C000272323

Contents

Foreword   v
Permissions   vi
Acknowledgements   vii
Introduction   ix

1   The History of the Practical Examination   1
2   The Examination   5
3   Anaesthesia   11
4   Bandaging   21
5   Fluid Therapy   37
6   Laboratory Techniques   49
7   Medical Nursing   73
8   Radiography   99
9   Surgical Nursing   127
10 Answers   143

Recommended Further Reading   147
Useful Addresses   151
Index   153

Foreword

Texts for student Veterinary Nurses have increased in number over the past few years, and now comprehensively cover a wide range of subjects. A whole variety of revision guides are available to assist the student VN in their preparation for the written examinations – but until now there has not been a single concise text that enables the reader to understand the practical examination process, from arrival at the Examination Centre to what to expect during the practical examination, and what to do if there are any problems before or during the examination process.

More importantly than this, for the first time this text also gives the reader an insight into what the examiners may be looking for, and the range of practical knowledge the student may be asked to show during the four different practical sets, all written to enable the reader to practise the necessary skills prior to the exams themselves.

Assessors and lecturers of student VNs will also find this a very useful guide in preparing mock examinations for their students, to make them as real-life as possible in the training practice or college.

This text has been written by a very experienced Veterinary Nurse, who is also an experienced RCVS Practical Examiner, and is a must for every student VN who is undergoing preparation for, what is, the most feared section of the examination process. I know because I can remember mine!

Lisa Cooper VN

Permissions

Image 6.2 (page 51) in this book is reproduced with permission from Elsevier from: *Clinical Procedures in Veterinary Nursing,* 2nd edition, Edited by Victoria Aspinall, 2003.

Image 7.1 (page 76) in this book is reproduced with permission from: *An Interpret Guide to Dog and Puppy Care,* 1987, published by Salamander books.

Image 9.1 (page 130) in this book is reproduced with permission from Elsevier from: *Berry and Kohn's Operating Room Technique,* 9th edition, 2000, Mosby.

Image 9.2 (page 131) in this book is reproduced with the permission of the BSAVA from: *Manual of Practical Veterinary Nursing,* edited by Simpson, 1994.

Acknowledgements

The author would like to thank the following people for their invaluable help in the writing of this book. The staff of The Bakewell Veterinary Centre in Derbyshire, and Moy Farm Veterinary Centre (in particular, Michelle Theobald) in Lancashire, for putting up with me always having my camera in my hand. Thanks to NationWide Laboratories, Lancashire for their help with the laboratory section pictures, also thanks to examiner Janis Hamilton and assistant examiner Lisa Jarvis for their constructive criticism for the laboratory section.

And to all Student Veterinary Nurses who gave me the idea of writing the book.

Introduction

The tasks candidates are expected to perform and complete for the Royal College of Veterinary Surgeons (RCVS) Practical Examination are all important nursing skills that should be performed competently and correctly by any qualified veterinary nurse (VN). The aim of the VN qualification is to enable candidates to enter any veterinary practice and be able to nurse safely. The practical examination verifies a nurse's ability to practise nursing safely. It is, therefore, vital that candidates practise these skills as often as possible.

This book is intended as a revision guide to help candidates practise the skills required to pass the practical examination. It should be used in collaboration with a sufficient knowledge of the subjects concerned, and a thorough understanding of the thought processes behind each task and question.

Chapter 1
The History of the Practical Examination

The practical section of the Veterinary Nursing Examination has been in place ever since the first Veterinary Nurses (or RANA's as they were then known) qualified back in 1963. Veterinary Nursing is a very practical subject and, as such, practical competence had to be demonstrated.

The Veterinary Nursing Examination has seen many changes since it was first implemented. At one stage, a practical examination was in place for both preliminary and final examinations. These practical exams were composed of two sections, an oral/viva section and a practical 'spotter' section. The oral/viva section was further split into four sections and the practical 'spotter' examination comprised 50 tasks/questions with 2 minutes allowed at each table. When the bell rang, every student had to stand up and move to the next question – it certainly put you under some pressure, even moving in the right direction proved difficult for some candidates. The dreaded 'spotter' examination is still used to test undergraduate veterinary surgeons today, although they call it the 'steeplechase'.

In 1996 the examination changed to become more structured. The preliminary and final examinations changed to Part I and Part II Examinations. Rather than a chat with an examiner who could probe your knowledge, a strict set of questions became the norm and no examiner was allowed to deviate from them. The first year practical examination was stopped; instead, the nurse would have to prove knowledge from both first and second years at the same time during the Part II Examination. This was used to ensure a standardised knowledge across the board. Students had to complete 3 tasks per section, a total of 12 tasks in $1^{1}/_{2}$ hours.

In 1999 Veterinary Nurse Training became a National Vocational Qualification (NVQ), or SNVQ if you resided in Scotland. The number of tasks dropped from 12 to just 8, but the time allowed per task remained the same, a total of 6 minutes was allowed per task. It has taken a few years for the old style examination to stop as many nurses fail the practical examination each and every year. This has given British-trained veterinary nurses the reputation of being amongst the best in the world. If the examination was easy, then the Veterinary Nurse qualification wouldn't mean as much as it does to so many nurses – we are proud to be Veterinary Nurses as we have worked so hard to pass the exams.

Currently NVQ level II is the first stage of the Veterinary Nursing Examination. This entails two $1^{1}/_{2}$ hour multiple choice examination papers. Provided your portfolio is complete, if you are successful at the level II exam, you progress to the level III exam. This also entails two $1^{1}/_{2}$ hour multiple choice papers, but, in addition to this, there is the practical section. You can't enrol for the level III examination until you have completed at least 60% of your portfolio. The Principal of your approved Training and Assessment Practice (or the Principal of the College where you are currently attending a residential course) has to sign a statement to prove that fact. Your Veterinary Nursing Approved Centre (VNAC) will be using your tracking records and if you haven't reached the 60%

mark, then you can be refused permission to sit the entire examination. This may seem harsh, but it has been proven that the nurses most likely to fail their level III examinations are those who have not achieved 60% of their portfolio. So, you are more likely to pass your practical examination if you have completed more than 60% of your portfolio when you apply for your level III examination.

During 2003 the re-accreditation of Veterinary Nursing qualifications was carried out by the Qualifications and Curriculum Authority (QCA). The Royal College of Veterinary Surgeons (RCVS) Level 2 and 3 syllabus and external written examinations are now accredited as qualifications in their own right. These qualifications will be known as Certificates in Small Animal Veterinary Nursing Theory and are also known as Vocationally Related Qualifications (VRQs). These VRQs still link closely with the NVQ system and the National Occupational Standards, and are for the written element of the examination only. All student Veterinary Nurses must now be provided with access to RCVS-approved courses of instruction, whether provided by an approved college or via formal in-house teaching that has been granted RCVS approval. From 2005, it is the course providers who will be required to submit external examination entries for their candidates and the results of the examinations will be sent to colleges and in-house teachers as well as individual candidates.

Chapter 2
The Examination

DO NOT FORGET YOUR CANDIDATE CARD!! – this is required to be shown to the examiner before every section commences. This card has your candidate number on it and this number stays with you throughout your written and practical examinations.

Give yourself plenty of time to arrive at your chosen examination centre. It may even be an idea to stop overnight somewhere close by so that you are fresh by the time you get to your examination centre, rather than in a crumpled heap having had problems with the journey and only just made it on time by the skin of your teeth. Arriving the night before will also give you time to familiarise yourself with the area, so you won't get lost with vital minutes to spare. You must arrive at your chosen examination centre 15 minutes before your practical examination start time. Failure to do so cannot guarantee that you will be granted entry into the examination, unless there has been a good reason for your delay. The examination timetable and other candidate requirements will take precedence.

Candidates must wear their uniform or protective clothing for the practical exam; this is for health and safety reasons. You will find, however, that wearing your uniform will have psychological advantages and you will be able to complete the task much more easily than if you were not in uniform. You are allowed to bring a calculator to the examination, although there will be one provided if the task requires a calculation to be performed. Maybe even bring your own scissors as you may reach for them subconsciously during the task if you are performing a bandaging procedure. Ensure long hair is tied back, any nail varnish is removed and you are not wearing jewellery before you arrive ready for your practical examination.

When you arrive at your chosen centre for your actual examination, you will be placed in groups of four. Each candidate is allocated to one of four examination rooms, and moves between rooms throughout the hour-long examination but is never in the same room as another candidate at the same time. As you arrive, you should be met by the senior examiner who will introduce himself/herself and brief you about the examination process. The senior examiner will go through the examination format again and let you know the names of the examiners for each section. They will explain about the assistant examiners and will let you know if the External Verifier will be present. If there is anything you don't understand at this stage, inform the senior examiner; chances are the other three candidates in your group will be in the same boat. After the briefing is complete, the examination will start.

The tasks

There are currently four sections to the practical oral examinations: radiography, laboratory, medical nursing and fluid therapy, and finally surgical nursing and anaesthesia. In each of the four sections there are two tasks lasting for a maximum of 6 minutes each.

Before you attempt the task, the examiner will show you the equipment you can use for the task. Everything you require to complete the task will be in front of you; if there is something you think is missing, then ask the examiner before grabbing at any other equipment that might be in the room. There is time allocated for you to read the task before starting it – make sure you read the task thoroughly and ask anything you do not understand. Once the timer has begun, think about the task in a logical manner and try to pretend that you are in your own practice. Nerves will be present on the day but, as in any performance, think about controlling them, rather than letting them take over. There will be an alarm that will sound after the first 4 minutes indicating that you will have 2 minutes remaining.

Oral questions

At the time of writing, oral questions are asked when the practical element of the examination has been completed, but this is to change. The examination is a practical one and passing it is based on your practical performance. Oral questions that may be asked during the practical examination have, therefore, been omitted from this book. There are many different questions that may be asked and it is beyond the limits of this book to predict which oral question you may be asked – besides, this book isn't here to help you cheat! So, don't rush through the task to get to the questions, because performing the task competently will gain you more marks than the oral questions alone. If you fail to complete the task, the examiner is not allowed to ask you the oral questions.

If you fly through the task and have minutes left after completing the questions as well, you cannot carry these minutes over to your next task to give you more time – it doesn't work like that. Once you have finished in one room, as you go through the door clear your mind ready for the next section – don't go over in your mind what you didn't do, as this will make you feel worse and lose your concentration for the next section.

For each task you are expected to perform, you have up to 6 minutes to prove your knowledge to the examiner. Despite the portfolio being a means of assessment, the tasks that you are expected to perform at the examinations all have important health and safety aspects for you, your colleagues and your patients. The examination is also an important method of ensuring that everyone meets the national occupational standards. This is why the examinations are still very much a necessity as a means of qualifying as a Veterinary Nurse. If the examination was easy, the qualification wouldn't mean as much as it does. Get an assessor in your practice to set up a mock examination and treat it like the real thing, then you will have even more experience of the procedure before the big day arrives.

Should your training practice not provide you with the chance to perform all of the required tasks, for example gloving and gowning, on a routine basis, talk to a neighbouring practice to see if they will let you 'see practice' there. This will enable you to practise these tasks whilst being supervised by people who carry them out daily.

Remember that at any given time on any given day every other student Veterinary Nurse up and down the country will be having the same task practical to perform. You will not be asked anything that a qualified Veterinary Nurse should not be able to perform. It is human nature, however, to go over everything you did wrong within the examination process and talk yourself into the fact that you have failed.

The examiners

Obviously there will be an examiner in the room with you when you perform these tasks, who is either a qualified Veterinary Nurse or Veterinary Surgeon. All have their assessing units, D32/33 or A1, so they are fully qualified to assess you. In addition, they have undergone further training to ensure they are competent RCVS assessors. So examiners are not monsters with three heads – they are just there to ensure the National Occupational Standard has been met. In addition to the examiner, there will be an assistant examiner in the room whilst you are completing your tasks. This person will also be either a qualified Veterinary Nurse or Veterinary Surgeon, but they are watching the fairness of the examination, ensuring that the examiner treats you no differently from other candidates, so don't think that there are lots of people staring at you. You can also use the assistant examiner if you require any help with anything, but obviously they cannot tell you the answers! Even though they are qualified Veterinary Nurses or Veterinary Surgeons, treat them as if they know nothing and let them know exactly what you want them to do. There may also be another person in the room, the External Verifier. Again, this person is there to oversee the fairness of the whole examination and to ensure that all candidates at each examination centre are treated fairly and equally, as they will travel from centre to centre within the same week.

Mitigating circumstances

There will be times when something does go wrong that is out of your hands; for example, a power cut during the examination. Try not to let it bother you, but carry on as you were doing. After the examination is complete, write down what happened and inform the RCVS. The assistant examiner will have documented anything abnormal during the examination anyway, but the abnormal event may have put you off further parts of the examination. You must inform the RCVS of any mitigating circumstances before the examination, or within five days of the practical examination if you think something happened to seriously affect your performance during the examination itself.

Chapter 3

Anaesthesia

Introduction

Anaesthesia is probably the most important aspect of your (a VN) day-to-day work. Even though the anaesthetic procedure is ultimately the responsibility of the Veterinary Surgeon, it is commonly your responsibility to prepare the anaesthetic equipment and to monitor the patient during anaesthesia and during their recovery. Inadequate knowledge could easily result in the death of a patient as their life is in your hands whilst they are anaesthetised.

What you need to know

Anaesthetic circuits and their characteristics

* You must be able to identify the Jackson Rees modified Ayre's T-piece, Magill, Bain and Lack (co-axial and/or parallel).
* Utilising the wrong circuit can have serious implications; at best it can cause premature awakening from anaesthesia, at worst it could cause patient death.

Safe circuit assembly

* You must be able to assemble the circuit for safe and effective use.
* Circuits may be disassembled for various reasons, eg cleaning and disinfection.

☙ Although the circuits we use are designed for one use only, they are rarely used only once in veterinary practice.

Safe working environment

☙ The scavenging tube must be attached to the circuit correctly, otherwise waste gases will escape into the atmosphere.
☙ Everyone has the right to work in a safe environment.

Safe practice

☙ You must correctly calculate the anaesthetic flow rate for the given circumstance.
☙ Inadequate flow rates can at best cause premature awakening of the patient – at worst they can cause brain damage.
☙ Circuit factors are numbers which allow you to be able to work out the correct flow rate to be employed. Each circuit works differently and this is illustrated by the circuit factors. A circuit with a factor of 3 needs 3 times more gas flow than a circuit with a factor of 1.

Table 3.1

Circuit Name	Factor
Magill	1 – 1.5
Parallel Lack/Co-axial Lack	1 – 1.5
Bains	2.5 – 3
Jackson Rees modified Ayres T-piece	2.5 – 3

☙ This chapter will show you how to work out the anaesthetic flow rate and examples for you to practise are given at the end of the chapter.

Intubation equipment and its use

- You must be able to choose the correct endotracheal tube and/or check the tube provided is safe for use.
- This tube is the patient's lifeline and must be in good working order before it is employed during anaesthesia.

Using anaesthetic equipment in practice

You are expected to be able to recognise the most suitable circuit for the patient and assemble it in the correct manner. Failure to do so could result in patient death.

Note: The scavenging valve on the circuit must be in the open position; otherwise, the patient's lungs will not be able to empty, having catastrophic results.

Circuits

You will come across a number of different anaesthetic circuits in practice:

The **Bain circuit** is recognised by the small green tube on the inside of the larger white corrugated tubing. The valve is together with the reservoir bag. The Bain circuit factor is 2.5–3.

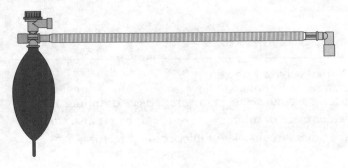

Figure 3.1   The Bain circuit

The **Magill** is recognised by the scavenging valve being separate from the reservoir bag. The Magill circuit factor is 1– 1.5.

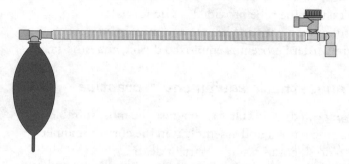

Figure 3.2   The Magill circuit

The **Parallel Lack** is recognised by two pieces of tubing of the same length, and by the distinctive double piece that connects to the anaesthetic machine. The reservoir bag connects underneath. The Lack circuit factor is 1– 1.5.

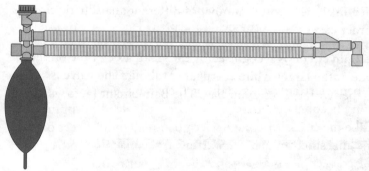

Figure 3.3   The Parallel Lack circuit

The **T-piece** is recognised by a long thin piece of tubing and a shorter wider piece of tubing. The reservoir bag is also smaller than in the other circuits. The T-piece circuit factor is 2.5–3.

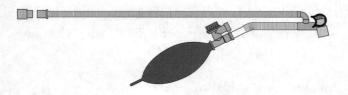

Figure 3.4 Jackson Rees modified T-piece

Circuit assembly

In order to be able to assemble the circuits correctly, you must have knowledge of what each type of circuit looks like and how it functions. In day to day practice, you must be able to:

* select the correct anaesthetic circuit
* assemble it correctly and attach it to the anaesthetic machine
* ensure the scavenging valve is in the open position
* attach the scavenging tube correctly
* check that the endotracheal tube provided is safe for use.

Practical tips

* When selecting and assembling the circuit, ensure the pieces don't become mixed up, as this can easily lead to confusion.
* Take the circuit you have selected and all of its pieces over to the anaesthetic machine. Starting at the machine end, attach the correct pieces and work towards your patient.

Calculation technique

You must be able to work out the gas flow rate needed for your patient. Remember, to calculate this, you must be able to recall the circuit factor for each circuit.

Example: Calculate the range of gas flow rates for a 15-kg dog with a respiratory rate of 15 breaths per minute, using a Magill circuit.

1 Work out the patient's tidal volume.
   - Depending on the patient's weight, a factor of 10 or 15 is used to discover the tidal volume.
   - For patients under 10 kg, use a tidal volume factor of 15; for patients weighing 10 kg and over, use a tidal volume factor of 10.
   - In this case the tidal volume is calculated as 15 kg × 10 ml/kg = 150 ml.

2 Calculate the patient's minute volume.
   - To do this, multiply the tidal volume (150 ml) by the respiratory rate (15 breaths per minute).
   - In this case, the minute volume is 150 ml × 15 breaths/min = 2250 ml/min.

3 Calculate the correct range of flow rates per minute.
   - To do this, multiply the minute volume (2250 ml) by the circuit factor (circuit factor for the Magill circuit is 1–1.5).
   - In this case, the flow rate is calculated as:
     2250 × 1 = 2250 ml or 2.25 litres
     2250 × 1.5 = 3375 ml or 3.37 litres.
   - Ensure that you include the range of flows, not just one flow rate. So, in this case, the range would be 2.25–3.37 litres.

Intubation

You must be able to select the most appropriate endotracheal tube size for a patient. You may need to select the appropriate tube from a selection of different-sized tubes, both cuffed and uncuffed. You should also be familiar with the depolarising neuromuscular blocking agents used to facilitate intubation and should be able to select the correct agent for the patient.

Quick test

Examples of anaesthetic calculations

(Answers on page 143)

1 Calculate the flow rate required for a 4.2-kg domestic shorthair cat using a Jackson Rees modified Ayre's T-piece. Assume the respiratory rate to be 20 breaths per minute.

. . . 3·3 8 litres . . . .

2 Calculate the flow rate required for a 9-kg Cavalier King Charles Spaniel using a Co-axial Lack circuit. Assume the respiratory rate to be 15 breaths per minute.

. 2025 - 3 038 litres . . . .

3 Calculate the flow rate required for a 5.2-kg domestic shorthair cat using a Jackson Rees modified Ayre's T-piece. Assume the respiratory rate to be 20 breaths per minute.

. 3·9 - 4·7 litres . . . . .

4 Calculate the flow rate required for a 6-kg Lhasa Apso using a Jackson Rees modified Ayre's T-piece. Assume the respiratory rate to be 20 breaths per minute.

. 4:5 - 5·4 litres . . . . . .

5 Calculate the flow rate required for a 28-kg Labrador using a Bain's circuit. Assume the respiratory rate to be 20 breaths per minute.

↗10

. . . 14 - 16·8 litres . . . .

6 Calculate the flow rate required for a 2.8-kg Persian using a Jackson Rees modified Ayre's T-piece. Assume the respiratory rate to be 15 breaths per minute.

↗15

. 1·6 - 1·9 litres . . . .

7 Calculate the flow rate required for a 4-kg cat using a Jackson Rees modified Ayre's T-piece. Assume the respiratory rate to be 20 breaths per minute.

↗15

. 3·3·6 litres . . . .

8 Calculate the flow rate required for a 32-kg dog using a Magill circuit. Assume the respiratory rate to be 15 breaths per minute.

↗10

. 4·8 - 7·2 litres . . . .

9 Calculate the flow rate for a 28-kg Border Collie using a Parallel Lack. Assume the respiratory rate to be 20 breaths per minute.

↗10

. 5·6 - 8·4 · litres . . . . . .

10 Calculate the flow rate for a 3.2-kg tortoiseshell cat using a Jackson Rees modified Ayre's T-piece. Assume the respiratory rate to be 15 breaths per minute.

↗15

. . . . 1·8 - 2·2 litres . . . .

↗10

11 Calculate the flow rate for an 18-kg Springer Spaniel using a Co-axial Lack circuit. Assume the respiratory rate to be 15 breaths per minute.

. . . 2·7 - 4·05 litres . . . . .

↗10

12 Calculate the flow rate for a 22-kg Labrador using a Bain's circuit. Assume the respiratory rate to be 20 breaths per minute.

. . 11 - 13·2 litres . . . .

↗10

13 Calculate the flow rate for a 35-kg Briard using a Parallel Lack circuit. Assume the respiratory rate to be 15 breaths per minute.

. 5·3 - 7·9 litres . . . . . .

↗10

14 Calculate the flow rate for a 16-kg crossbred dog using a Magill circuit. Assume the respiratory rate to be 20 breaths per minute.

. . 3·2 - 4·8 litres . . . . .

ANAESTHESIA

Chapter 4
Bandaging

Introduction

You should be proficient in applying all types of bandage, whether it is for the thorax, a foot or an ear. Very often, it is the VN who is given responsibility for bandage application and aftercare. Bandages can be applied for various reasons – pressure, support, immobilisation and protection.

What you need to know

Bandaging materials

* You must have sound knowledge of the different types of wound dressings and bandaging materials.
* There are hundreds of types available and it is imperative that you are proficient in their use.

Health and safety

* You must have a sound understanding of health and safety and be able to apply this knowledge when bandaging.
* Any conscious patient must be restrained by an assistant prior to any bandaging attempt, otherwise serious injury could occur.

Safe bandaging technique

The general rules to be followed when bandaging include:

21

- You must be able to demonstrate that you are able to apply any bandage correctly and proficiently
- Always start with clean hands
- Always collect materials together before use and keep them all within easy reach
- Ensure the patient is restrained by an assistant in a safe and appropriate manner
- Ensure that the area to be bandaged has been identified correctly
- Always remove and dispose of soiled dressings
- Where appropriate, apply a suitable wound dressing in a sterile manner over the wound.
- Always ensure you use the correct type of bandage
- Always enclose foot if bandaging a lower limb
- Always pad pressure points
- Always begin distal to proximal when bandaging limbs
- Always unroll a small amount of bandage at one time
- Always apply with even tension
- Always apply with spiral action, giving 1/2 to 2/3 overlap
- Always avoid sticking the bandage to the patient's fur
- Always include the joint above and below when bandaging a fracture
- Apply synthetic cast padding over an area to be splinted, to avoid direct contact between the splint and the patient's fur
- Ensure the bandage is neat and comfortable

Safe practice

- You must have a sound understanding of what constitutes a safe bandage and what constitutes an unsafe bandage.
- An incorrectly applied bandage can be detrimental to the patient and cause major problems.
- A bandage must be able to perform its function, otherwise there is no point in applying it.

Aftercare

❧ Frequently, you will need to discuss bandage aftercare with clients.

❧ It is most important to show confidence and knowledge when talking to owners.

Practical tips

You must be able to apply bandages proficiently. Irreparable damage can be caused by inappropriate bandage application: too loose and the bandage may fall off; too tight and it may restrict breathing or the patient may interfere with it. Patients have been known to require limb amputation following the incorrect application of bandages. Patients usually require restraint before bandages are applied.

You must be able to select the appropriate bandaging technique in a given clinical situation. You should know when to apply conforming, cohesive and non-cohesive bandages, and also how many layers should be applied. You should also be able to select the correct sized splint, where applicable.

The following case studies are helpful illustrations of what to do in practice.

Case Study 1

The Robert Jones bandage applied to support an internally fixed, fractured left radius and ulna

Practical tips

- ❦ Ensure the patient is restrained by an assistant in a safe and appropriate manner with the affected limb uppermost. Ensure you are going to bandage the correct limb.
- ❦ Place stirrups either on the dorsal and caudal aspect of the limb or on the medial and lateral aspect depending on where the wound is – don't cover the wound with the stirrups.
- ❦ Pad the toes with cotton wool.
- ❦ Apply an appropriate wound dressing to the wound in a sterile manner.
- ❦ Apply cotton wool to the limb straight from the roll, applying at least four layers. The bandage should allow the two central toes to be visible, and extend over the elbow.
- ❦ Starting at the distal aspect of the limb, apply conforming bandage under sufficient tension to compress the cotton wool.
- ❦ Once the entire length of cotton wool is compressed, then reflect back the stirrups and stick them to the conforming bandage underneath, again to ensure you can still see the two central toes.
- ❦ Apply a tertiary layer, with either adhesive or cohesive bandage, and again start at the distal end and work proximally.
- ❦ Ensure the bandage is neat and comfortable.

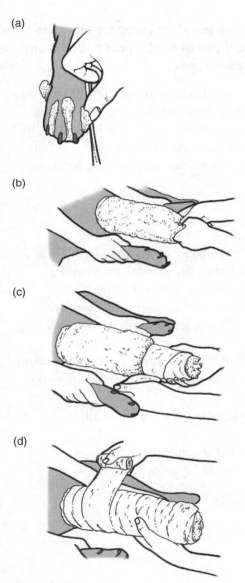

Figure 4.1 (a) Dog's paws with cotton wool between toes and 'stirrups' being placed on either side; (b) Dog's leg being covered with cotton wool; (c) Cotton wool being compressed using conforming bandage; (d) Outer layer being applied

Case Study 2

Bandage the right forepaw after the surgical removal of a grass seed from its dorsal aspect

You must be able to apply this bandage proficiently. Applying a foot bandage too tightly may cause the patient to interfere with the bandage, which could be detrimental. Apply it too loosely and it will probably fall off. Adequate restraint of the patient must be performed before you attempt to place this bandage.

Practical tips

Bandage technique

- Ensure the patient is restrained by an assistant in a safe and appropriate manner with the affected limb uppermost. Ensure you are going to bandage the correct limb.
- Pad between the toes with small amounts of cotton wool.
- Apply a suitable wound dressing in a sterile manner over the wound.
- Starting at the distal tip of the foot, apply either cotton wool or synthetic cast padding over the limb, extending over the carpus.
- Apply conforming bandage, again starting distally and working proximally.
- Apply the tertiary layer in the same manner.
- Ensure the bandage is neat and comfortable.

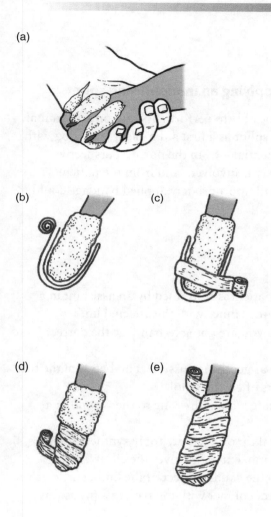

Figure 4.2 (a) Cotton wool placed between toes; (b) conforming bandage applied to the dorsal and palmar aspect of the paw; (c), (d), (e) wrap conforming bandage around the paw, moving in a distal to proximal manner

3 Applying an immobilising splint

Case Study

You are expected to be able to perform first aid on any animal. Being able to apply a splint as a first aid measure to a dog with a fractured limb is essential – from the nurse's perspective where health and safety is involved, and from the patient's perspective where an ill-appropriately applied bandage could prove detrimental.

Practical tips

Bandage technique

- Again, ensure the patient is restrained by an assistant in a safe and appropriate manner with the affected limb uppermost. Ensure you are going to bandage the correct limb.
- Handling the limb as gently as possible, pad between the toes with small amounts of cotton wool.
- Apply an appropriate wound dressing to the wound in a sterile manner.
- Starting at the distal tip of the foot, apply synthetic cast padding over the limb, extending over the elbow.
- Apply the splint to the caudal aspect of the limb, ensuring the splint is not in direct contact with the patient's fur as this would rub.
- Starting at the distal tip of the foot, apply conforming bandage over the limb and splint, and extending over the elbow.
- Apply the tertiary layer in the same manner.
- Ensure the bandage is neat and comfortable.

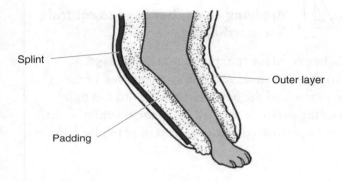

Figure 4.3   Cross-section of a correctly applied splint

Case Study

4 Applying an ear bandage to control haemorrhaging

You should be proficient at applying an ear bandage, as improper application could result in strangulation of the patient. Too loose and the bandage will slip off, too tight and it will constrict the patient's airway. Adequate restraint of the patient must be performed before you attempt to place this bandage.

Practical tips

Bandage technique

- Again, ensure the patient is restrained by an assistant in a safe and appropriate manner.
- Place a small pad of cotton wool on top of the patient's ear.
- Cover the ear tip in a sterile manner with an appropriate wound dressing.
- Reflect the ear over the top of the patient's head.
- Apply padding over the ear and under the chin.
- Apply conforming bandage over the ear and under the chin. Use a figure of eight pattern using the healthy ear as an anchor.
- Apply cohesive bandage in the same manner.
- Check the bandage is neat and is not too tight, check the patient can see and that they can also open their mouth.

(a)

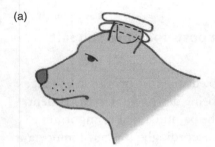

(b)

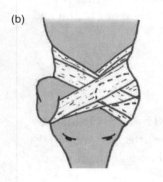

(c)

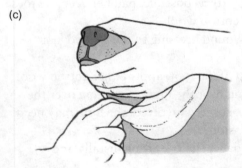

Figure 4.4 Applying an ear bandage. (a) Affected ear reflected on top of head with padding in place; (b) figure-of-eight, anchoring bandage into position; (c) checking to ensure bandage is not too tight or too loose

BANDAGING

Case Study

5

Applying a post-operative support bandage

It is often your responsibility to ensure post-operative bandages are applied correctly, without being detrimental to the patient. Post-operatively, the area will be painful and it is important to ensure the patient is dealt with accordingly. It is most important that this patient is restrained correctly before starting your bandage. Failure to do so could compromise your health and safety.

Practical tips

Bandage technique

- Again, ensure the patient is restrained by an assistant in a safe and appropriate manner with the affected limb uppermost. Ensure you are going to bandage the correct limb.
- Handling the limb as gently as possible, pad between the toes with small amounts of cotton wool.
- Apply an appropriate wound dressing to the wound in a sterile manner.
- Starting at the distal tip of the foot, apply either cotton wool or synthetic cast padding over the limb, extending over the stifle. Depending on the surgery involved, the limb may need to be bandaged in extension.
- Apply conforming bandage, again starting distally and working proximally.
- Apply the tertiary layer in the same manner.
- Ensure the bandage is neat and comfortable.

Please see Figure 4.2 in Case study 2 for further guidance.

Case Study

Applying a Robert Jones bandage to support a compound-fractured right radius and ulna

You must be able to apply this bandage proficiently. Irreparable damage can be caused by inappropriate bandage application. Patients have been known to require limb amputation following the incorrect application of this bandage. Reasons for the application of this bandage include first aid support following a lower limb fracture, to reduce swelling and pain.

Practical tips

Bandage technique

- 🐾 Again, ensure the patient is restrained by an assistant in a safe and appropriate manner with the affected limb uppermost. Ensure you are going to bandage the correct limb.
- 🐾 Place the stirrups on the dorsal and caudal aspect of the limb – don't cover the wound with the stirrups.
- 🐾 Pad between the toes with cotton wool.
- 🐾 Apply an appropriate wound dressing to the wound in a sterile manner.
- 🐾 Apply cotton wool to the limb straight from the roll, applying at least four layers. The bandage should allow the two central toes to be visible, and extend over the elbow.
- 🐾 Starting at the distal aspect of the limb, apply conforming bandage under sufficient tension to compress the cotton wool.
- 🐾 Once the entire length of cotton wool is compressed, then reflect back the stirrups and stick them to the conforming bandage underneath, again to ensure you can still see the two central toes.

- Apply a tertiary layer, with either adhesive or cohesive bandage, and again start at the distal end and work proximally.
- Ensure the bandage is neat and comfortable.

Please see Figure 4.1 in Case study 1 for further guidance.

Case Study

7 Applying a thoracic bandage to a dog who has a wound over the manubrium

Thoracic bandages are used to cover wounds, to cover drains or to prevent wound interference. You must be proficient in their application as, if incorrectly applied, they could be detrimental to the patient. Too loosely applied and they could simply slip; too tightly applied and they could restrict the patient's breathing. You must ensure that the patient is adequately restrained before attempting this task, otherwise you may be bitten.

Practical tips

Bandage technique

* Again, ensure the patient is restrained by an assistant in a safe and appropriate manner.
* Apply a sterile wound dressing in a sterile manner over the wound.
* Using the synthetic cast padding, start the bandage over the scapula (point a) and go around the thorax until you meet the start of the bandage (point a). Then take the bandage over the shoulder and through the front legs and back up the other side of the thorax until you reach point a. Go around the thorax again but this time bring the bandage up through the front legs, back to point a. This should result in a 'figure of eight' pattern around the thorax, using the front legs as an anchor.
* Using the conforming bandage, repeat in the same manner as for the synthetic cast padding.
* Apply the tertiary layer in the same manner as above.
* Ensure the bandage is not too tight and that it is neat and comfortable.

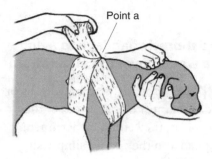

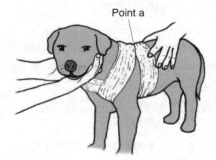

Figure 4.5   Applying a thoracic bandage

Chapter 5
Fluid Therapy

Introduction

Fluid therapy is an area of veterinary nursing that can be very rewarding. Various medical conditions can give rise to the need for fluid therapy, and the VN must be proficient in many areas of fluid therapy, from the selection of the correct equipment, to placing the intravenous catheter, through to observing the patient during fluid delivery. A patient can be over-infused as well as under-infused with detrimental results.

What you need to know

Types of intravenous fluid

* You must know when to use a crystalloid solution or whole blood, depending on the task in question.
* Giving a patient the wrong fluid could have serious, if not fatal, consequences.

Knowledge of equipment

* You must be able to identify and select the appropriate equipment for a procedure.
* Different equipment is needed according to the fluid required by the patient.
* Using the wrong equipment can have serious results and may cause patient fatalities.

Safe practical technique

* You must be able to correctly and safely prepare infusion equipment with due regard for asepsis.
* The equipment used in fluid therapy is designed to place fluid into the animal's circulatory system; with inadequate regard for asepsis, you could also introduce bacteria which would be detrimental to your patient.

Safe practice

* Your calculations must be correct: animals can quickly die or at least deteriorate with either inadequate or excessive fluid.
* As a VN, you will be expected to know how to monitor the drip rate and alter it according to the patient's requirements.
* Fluid therapy is a dynamic process and, as such, the patient's needs could change continuously.
* Examples of fluid therapy calculations for you to practise are given at the end of the chapter.

Types of intravenous catheter

* You must be able to select intravenous catheters of a suitable type and size for the given circumstances.
* An incorrect-sized catheter can damage the vein wall and make future intravenous catheterisations much more difficult to perform.

Assembly technique

* Tip: always check packets to ensure they are in date and discard any that are expired; however, in an exam situation, inform the examiner if they have expired but continue as though they are usable.

* Remove the fluid bag from the outer layer and suspend from infusion stand.
* Open any ports necessary, but don't touch the inside of them.
* Remove the packaging from the administration set and turn the controller off; ensure you leave the cap on both ends.
* Remove the cover from the spike on the giving set.
* Ensuring you do not touch the spike, push it into the port on the fluid bag.
* Keep pushing until the spike is correctly seated within the fluid bag.
* Squeeze the drip chamber to half fill it with fluid.
* SLOWLY open the controller to allow fluid to run through the line to the end.
* Suspend the primed administration line over the drip stand ready for use.

See Figure 5.1 overleaf.

Practical tips

You must be able to calculate the fluid therapy requirements of the patient. First, you must select the correct equipment for placing an intravenous catheter and place this equipment to one side. Next you must assemble the fluid bag and administration set ready for use. Then, you must calculate the fluid therapy regime for your patient.

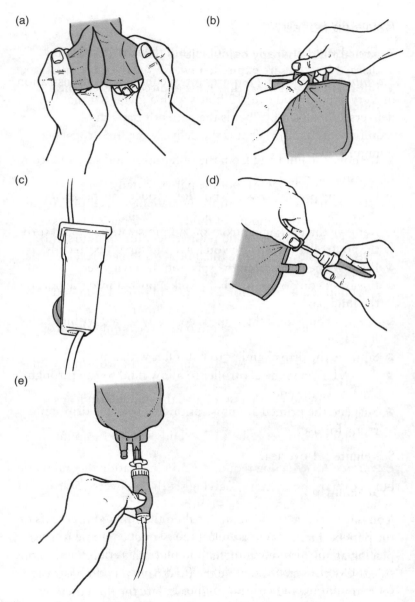

Figure 5.1 Drip assembly. (a) Remove packaging; (b) open port; (c) close controller; (d) insert spike; (e) squeeze chamber to half full. *Image courtesy of AQUPHARM from Animalcare*

Revision notes

Practice fluid therapy calculations

Example: An x-kg dog requires intravenous (iv) administration of a crystalloid fluid over 12 hours with a giving set that delivers 20 drops/ml. What is the patient's daily fluid requirement (in ml)? What is the delivery rate (in drops) per minute?

1 First we need to work out the patient's daily fluid requirements in ml. Multiply the patient's weight by 50 ml (50 ml/kg is the amount of fluid required per 24 hours):
   - x kg × 50 ml/kg = fluid requirement for 24 hours (ml).
2 Divide this by 12 to give the fluid requirement rate over the 12 hours:
   - Fluid requirement for 24 hours (in ml) ÷ 12 (in hours) = fluid requirement per hour (ml/hour).
3 Multiply this by 20 drops/ml to give the number of drops per hour:
   - Fluid requirement (in ml/hour) × 20 (in drops/ml) = fluid drops per hour.
4 Divide this number by 60 to give the number of drops per minute:
   - Fluid drops per hour ÷ 60 = fluid drops per minute.

Example: An x-kg dog requires iv administration of y ml whole blood over 12 hours using a giving set that delivers 15 drops/ml. What is the drip rate in drops/min?

1 First we divide the amount of blood (y, in ml) by 12 hours to give the blood requirement in ml per hour:
   - Blood amount (y, in ml) ÷ 12 (in hours) = blood requirement per hour (ml/hour).
2 Divide this by 60 to give the blood requirement in ml per minute:

- Blood requirement per hour ÷ 60 = blood requirement (in ml/min).

3 Multiply this number by 15 drops/ml to give the blood drops per minute:
  - Blood requirement (in ml/min) × 15 (in drops/ml) = drip rate (in drops/min).

Example: An x-kg cat requires iv administration of a crystalloid fluid over y hours, with a giving set that delivers at z drops per ml. What is the drop rate needed to fulfill the maintenance requirements per day (in drops/min)?

1 First, work out the patient's daily fluid requirements (50 ml/kg per 24 hours):
  - 50 ml × x (in kg) = fluid requirement (in ml) for 24 hours.

2 Divide this by the number of hours over which the fluid is to be administered:
  - Fluid requirement for 24 hours (in ml) ÷ y (in hours) = fluid requirement per hour (in ml/hour).

3 Multiply this by the number of drops per ml:
  - Fluid requirement (in ml/hour) × z (in drops/ml) = fluid drop rate (in drops/hour).

4 Divide this number by 60 to give the drops per minute:
  - Fluid drops per hour ÷ 60 = fluid drops per minute.

Example: Calculate maintenance requirements for a 20-kg dog per day in ml. The volume of fluid calculated is to be given over 12 hours. What is the rate (in drops) per minute if the giving set delivers 20 drops/ml?

1 First we need to calculate the patient's daily fluid requirement in ml.

2 Multiply the patient's weight by 50 ml (50 ml/kg per day is the fluid requirement):
  - 20 kg × 50 ml/kg = 1000 ml fluid per day.

3 Divide this figure by 12 hours to give the fluid requirement per hour:
- 1000 ml ÷ 12 hours = 83 ml fluid requirement per hour.

4 Multiply this figure by 20 to give the number of drops per hour:
- 83 ml/hour × 20 drops/ml = 1667 drops/hour.

5 Divide this number by 60 to give the number of drops per minute:
- 1667 ÷ 60 = 28 drops per minute.

6 So the patient's maintenance requirements are 1000 ml of fluid per day at a rate of 28 drops per minute.

Example: 500 ml of whole blood is to be given to a 30-kg dog over 12 hours. Calculate the drip rate in ml/min and the drip rate in drops/min (the giving set delivers 15 drops/ml).

1 We already know the amount of fluid to be administered this time.

2 Divide this amount by 12 hours to get the volume of blood (in ml/hour) to be delivered:
- 500 ml ÷ 12 hours = 42 ml/hour.

3 Divide this number by 60 to give the number of ml per minute:
- 42 ÷ 60 = 0.7 ml/min.

4 Multiply this number by 15 to give the number of drops per minute:
- 0.7 ml/min × 15 drops/ml = 10.5 drops/min.

5 So the patient requires 0.7 ml of blood per minute, which is a rate of 10.5 drops per minute.

Example: Calculate maintenance requirements for a 4-kg cat per day in ml. The volume of fluid calculated is to be given over 24 hours. What is the rate (in drops) per minute if the giving set delivers 60 drops/ml?

1 First we need to calculate the patient's daily fluid requirement in ml.

2 Multiply the patient's weight by 50 ml (50 ml/kg per day is the fluid requirement):
  • 4 kg × 50 ml/kg = 200 ml fluid per day.
3 Divide this figure by 24 hours to give the fluid requirement per hour:
  • 200 ml ÷ 24 hours = 8 ml fluid requirement per hour.
4 Multiply this figure by 60 drops/ml to give the number of drops per hour:
  • 8 ml/hour × 60 drops/ml = 480 drops/hour.
5 Divide this number by 60 to give the number of drops per minute:
  • 480 ÷ 60 = 8 drops per minute.
6 So the patient's maintenance requirements are 200 ml of fluid per day at a rate of 8 drops per minute.

Quick test

(Answers on page 143)

Calculate the fluid therapy rates for the following patients

1 Calculate maintenance requirements for a 3.5-kg cat per day in ml. The volume of fluid calculated is to be given over 12 hours. What is the rate (in drops) per minute if the giving set delivers 60 drops/ml?

. 175ml per day. 15 drops. .

2 400 ml of whole blood is to be given to a 14-kg dog over 12 hours.
  a. Calculate the drip rate in ml/min.
  b. Calculate the drip rate in drops/min (the giving set delivers 15 drops/ml).

. 0.6ml . 18 drops/min . . .

3 Calculate maintenance requirements for a 25-kg dog per day in ml. The volume of fluid calculated is to be given over 24 hours. What is the rate (in drops) per minute if the giving set delivers 20 drops/ml?

1250 ml . / 17 drops / min.

4 Calculate maintenance requirements for a 2.5-kg cat per day in ml. The volume of fluid calculated is to be given over 12 hours. What is the rate (in drops) per minute if the giving set delivers 60 drops/ml?

125 ml / 10 drops / min .

5 500 ml of whole blood is to be given to a 27-kg dog over 12 hours.
a. Calculate the drip rate in ml/min.
b. Calculate the drip rate in drops/min (the giving set delivers 15 drops/ml).

0.7 ml / min . / 10 drops/min

6 Calculate maintenance requirements for a 12-kg dog per day in ml. The volume of fluid calculated is to be given over 12 hours. What is the rate (in drops) per minute if the giving set delivers 20 drops/ml?

600 ml / 17 drops/ min . .

7 Calculate maintenance requirements for a 2.7-kg cat per day in ml. The volume of fluid calculated is to be given over 12 hours. What is the rate (in drops) per minute if the giving set delivers 60 drops/ml?

135ml. / 11 drops/min

8 350 ml of whole blood is to be given to a 10-kg dog over 12 hours.
a. Calculate the drip rate in ml/min.
b. Calculate the drip rate in drops/min (the giving set delivers 15 drops/ml).

0.5ml.min. / 7 drops

9 Calculate maintenance requirements for an 8-kg dog per day in ml. The volume of fluid calculated is to be given over 24 hours. What is the rate (in drops) per minute if the giving set delivers 20 drops/ml?

400ml / 7 drops/min

10 Calculate maintenance requirements for a 5-kg cat per day in ml. The volume of fluid calculated is to be given over 12 hours. What is the rate (in drops) per minute if the giving set delivers 60 drops/ml?

250 ml / 21 drops/min

11 500 ml of whole blood is to be given to a 12-kg dog over
24 hours.
a. Calculate the drip rate in ml/min.
b. Calculate the drip rate in drops/min (the giving set
delivers 15 drops/ml).

0.35ml. / 5. drops/.min

12 Calculate maintenance requirements for a 35-kg dog per
day in ml. The volume of fluid calculated is to be given over
24 hours. What is the rate (in drops) per minute if the giving
set delivers 20 drops/ml?

1750ml / 24 drops/min

13 Calculate maintenance requirements for a 2-kg cat per day
in ml. The volume of fluid calculated is to be given over
24 hours. What is the rate (in drops) per minute if the giving
set delivers 60 drops/ml?

100 ml/. 4. drops/min.

Chapter 6
Laboratory Techniques

Introduction

Laboratory tests are used to aid or confirm a diagnosis made by the Veterinary Surgeon, and a patient's condition could easily be misdiagnosed if the test is performed incorrectly. You need to be familiar with the equipment in the laboratory, as you will be called upon to perform simple yet vital procedures in a veterinary practice. Some of the tasks could be utilised in an emergency and you will need to act proficiently, competently and safely whilst performing them. Details of many laboratory tests encountered in daily practice are given in the case studies later in this chapter.

What you need to know

Health and safety

This is an important aspect of working in the laboratory and as such some simple rules must be known and obeyed:

* Protective clothing must be worn when dealing with samples.
* Long hair must be tied back.
* No eating, drinking or smoking is allowed in the laboratory.
* Clinical waste, sharps and glass must be disposed of correctly.
* The laboratory coat must not be worn outside the laboratory.
* Hands must be washed prior to leaving the laboratory.

Proficient microscope use

* There are many different types of microscope, although they all have the same basic features. Help in using microscopes properly is given later in this chapter.

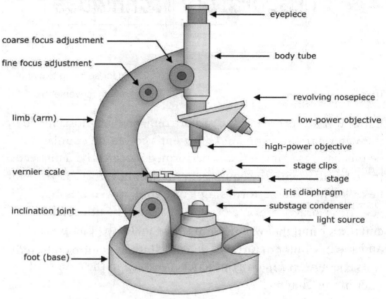

Figure 6.1   Microscope

Knowledge of vernier scales

* You must be able to locate the specimen on the prepared slide and identify the vernier scale reading. Full details are given in the Revision Notes at the end of the chapter.
* The vernier scale enables you to relocate an item on a slide should the slide be removed from the microscope, which will save time and effort if the item was difficult to find initially.
* There are some examples of vernier scale reading for you to practise at the end of this section.

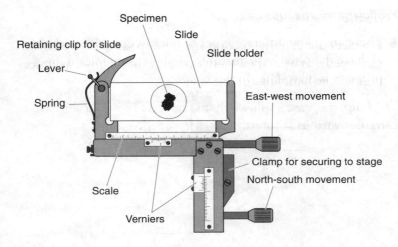

Figure 6.2 Vernier scale

Sample collection

🐾 This is often the role of the VN and you must know how samples of blood, fur, tissue, urine, faeces, etc are collected and stored to prevent sample deterioration.

Practical techniques

🐾 You must be able to prepare the sample for tests to be performed, and carry out certain tests.

Common parasites and their characteristics

🐾 You must correctly identify common parasites, know whether it is an ectoparasite or an endoparasite and give its correct name.

Common urine crystals and their characteristics

🐾 As the VN, you will often be asked to examine urine samples and so knowledge of how this is performed is vital.

Correct packaging techniques

🐾 Practices use external laboratories and so samples need to be packaged up correctly with due respect for the postal service that will be handling the specimen.

The following case studies help to illustrate how you should carry out various laboratory tasks in practice.

Urinary sediment examination

You are expected to be able to perform a urinary sediment examination competently and efficiently. Failure to do so could result in the inability to find signs of urinary problems in a patient, eg urine crystals. Cats in particular can suffer from urinary problems caused by Feline Urological Syndrome (FUS) and this can become life threatening if their urethra becomes blocked. You must also be able to prepare samples and use a microscope proficiently.

Practical tips

Preparing the sample

- Put on the gloves.
- Remove most of the supernatant fluid from the centrifuged sample using a pipette, being careful not to disturb the sediment.
- Resuspend the sample by tapping it with your fingers.
- Add a drop of Sedistain® to the sample (optional).
- Using a pipette, place a drop of the sample onto a microscope slide.
- Apply a coverslip carefully to avoid any air bubbles.

LABORATORY TECHNIQUES

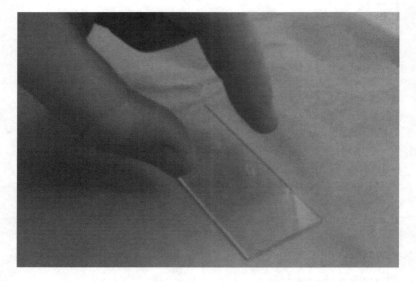

Figure 6.3   Cover slip placement on a microscope slide

Microscopic examination

* Place the slide on the microscope stage and secure it in place.
* Switch on the microscope.
* Examine the slide using the lowest objective lens (usually ×10).
* Find a crystal and focus on it using the coarse focus controls then the fine focus controls.
* Once it is in focus, change the objective lens to ×40.
* Place the crystal in the centre of your field of view, by making minor adjustments to the direction controls and fine focus.
* Identify the crystal and write down the vernier scale reading (*see* Revision notes for correct way to read the vernier scale).

Ensure that you are familiar with the crystals that can be found in either a dog's or cat's urine. They are pictured here for reference.

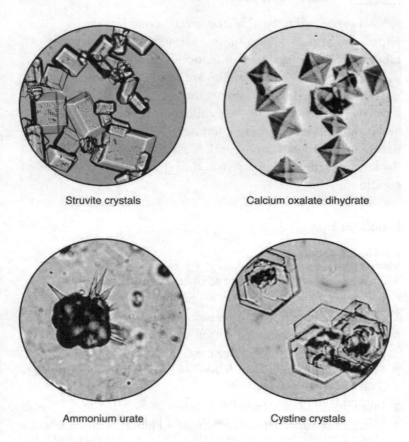

Struvite crystals

Calcium oxalate dihydrate

Ammonium urate

Cystine crystals

Figure 6.4   Urine crystals under microscope. *Images courtesy of Nova Professional Media.*

LABORATORY TECHNIQUES

Case Study 2 Packaging and labelling a histology sample

A VN is expected to be able to correctly complete the paperwork and package a sample for posting to a relevant laboratory. Histological examination is rarely performed in veterinary practices and samples are routinely dispatched to outside laboratories. Pathology samples are potentially hazardous to members of the public (post office workers, etc), and postal services can refuse improperly labelled or packaged pathology samples. Careful packaging also reduces sample damage and allows it to arrive at the laboratory in an unspoiled condition.

Practical tips

Packaging technique

* Ensure the screw lid on the sample container is fully tightened.
* Ensure the patient's name is written on the container.
* Wrap the tube in enough cotton wool to soak up all of the sample should the container break or leak.
* Place this in a sealable leak-proof plastic bag and ensure the bag is sealed correctly.
* Place the bag in a padded envelope.
* Mark the padded envelope 'Fragile – Handle with Care' using pen.
* Mark the padded envelope 'pathological specimen' using pen.
* Mark the back of the padded envelope with the practice name and address in pen.
* Complete the laboratory form correctly with the appropriate details in pen; for example:

Patient: 'Jackie' three-year-old cross-bred bitch
Owner: Mrs Jones, 4 The Park, Deal, BS3 4QR
Sample: a mammary gland
Lab: A.B. SERVICES, 1 High Street, Chigley, CB3 1KP
Vet: J. Smith, 2 High Road, Deal, BS4 2JP.

* Place the form in the envelope but not in the plastic bag.
* Seal the envelope with tape.

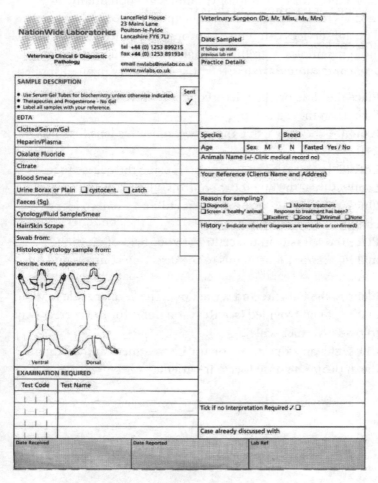

Figure 6.5   Lab form. *Courtesy of Nationwide Laboratories.*

Ectoparasite identification

It is often your responsibility to examine microscope slides to try to find ectoparasites. It is vital that you perform this competently and correctly, otherwise misdiagnosis may occur. A proficient microscope technique is required, as is a sound knowledge of parasites and their treatment.

Practical tips

Microscopic examination

- Place the slide on the microscope stage and secure it in place.
- Switch on the microscope.
- Examine the slide using the lowest objective lens (usually ×10).
- Locate the parasite and focus on it using the coarse focus controls then the fine focus controls.
- Once it is in focus, if the image is still too small to identify, change the objective lens to ×40.
- Place the parasite in the centre of your field of view by making minor adjustments to the direction controls and fine focus.
- Identify the parasite and write down the vernier scale reading on the paper provided (*see* Revision notes for the correct way to read a vernier scale).
- Chose the appropriate ectoparasite treatment and calculate the appropriate dose for your patient.

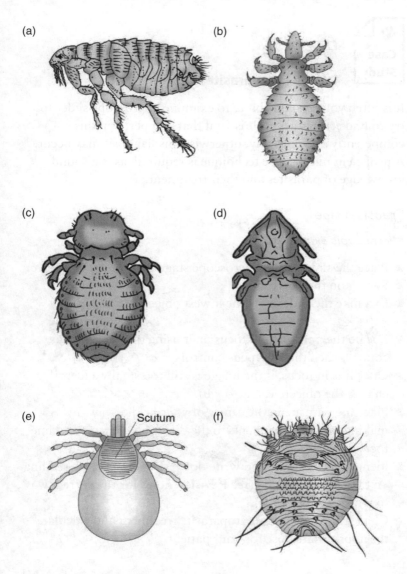

Figure 6.6 Ectoparasites: (a) *Ctenocephalides felis*; (b) *Linognathus setosus*; (c) *Trichodectes canis*; (d) *Felicola subrostratus*; (e) *Ixodes* spp.; (f) *Sarcoptes scabiei*

continues overleaf

(g)

(h)

(i)

Suckers

(j)

(k)

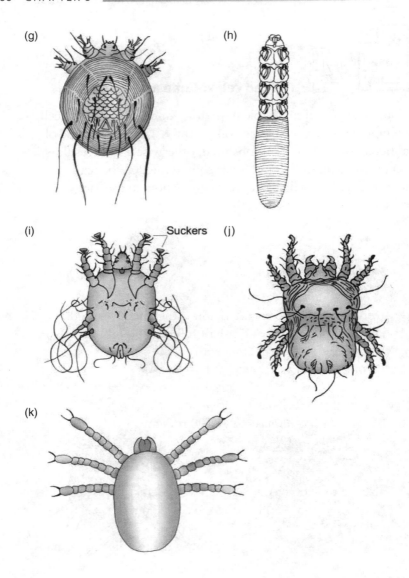

Figure 6.6   *Continued*
(g) *Notoedres cati*; (h) *Demodex canis*; (i) *Otodectes cynotis*; (j) *Cheyletiella* mite;
(k) *Trombicula autumnalis* larva

Case Study 4

Packed cell volume measurement

You are expected to be able to perform and read a packed cell volume (PCV) correctly and competently. The correct type of anticoagulated blood must be used, otherwise a false result will occur. Misdiagnosis could occur should the PCV be read incorrectly. You will also need to know how to use the centrifuge safely and correctly.

Practical tips

Preparing a PCV

- Put on the gloves.
- Invert the sample to ensure that it is thoroughly mixed.
- Fill two capillary tubes over half full with blood.
- Wipe the outside of the tube with tissue.
- Seal one end of each tube with Cristaseal™.
- Place the two tubes in the centrifuge opposite each other to balance it out, sealed end outwards.
- Centrifuge for 5 minutes at 10000 revs/min.

Reading a PCV (method 1)

- Place the tube on to the Hawksley™ haematocrit reader.
- Place the bottom of the red blood cell column on the baseline of the reader.
- Move the tube along the reader until the top of the plasma is level with the sloping line.
- Adjust the movable line until it is level with the top of the red blood cell column.
- Read the percentage value on the scale.

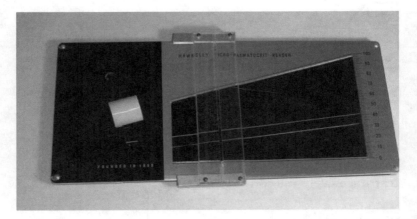

Figure 6.7 Haematocrit reader

Reading a PCV (method 2)

- ☙ Measure the length of the red blood cells (A).
- ☙ Measure the total length of the red blood cells, buffy coat and plasma (B).
- ☙ Divide (A) by (B).
- ☙ Multiply your result by 100 to get a percentage.

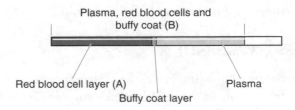

Figure 6.8 Measurements of PCV tube

Urine sample processing

You must be able to perform a specific gravity and dipstick test on urine in a correct and competent manner, otherwise misdiagnosis could occur. The refractometer must be carefully calibrated before each use to ensure the urine specific gravity results are accurate.

Practical tips

Refractometer technique

- Wipe the glass prism with tissue.
- Using a pipette, place distilled water onto the prism, enough to just cover it.
- Close the cover.
- Hold the refractometer up to the light and look at the correct scale through the eyepiece.
- If the reading is not exactly 1.000, adjust the screw at the top of the refractometer until the reading is exactly 1.000.
- Wipe the glass prism with tissue to remove the distilled water.
- Put on gloves.
- Invert the urine sample to ensure it is thoroughly mixed.
- Using a fresh pipette, place urine onto the prism, enough to just cover it.
- Close the cover.
- Hold the refractometer up to the light and read the scale as before.
- Wipe the prism clean with a tissue.
- Rinse the prism with distilled water and again wipe dry with a tissue.
- Record your results on paper.

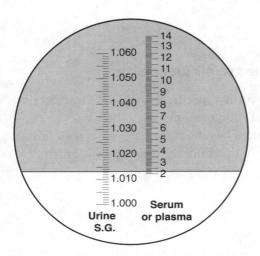

Figure 6.9 Scale reading (This reading equals a specific gravity of 1.013.)

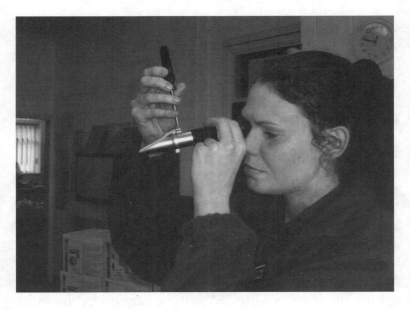

Figure 6.10 Calibrating refractometer

Dipstick technique

- 🐾 Select the appropriate urine dipstick and read the instructions on the label.
- 🐾 Check the expiry date on the chosen dipsticks.
- 🐾 Put gloves on.
- 🐾 Remove the dipstick test lid and remove one test stick.
- 🐾 Replace the lid.
- 🐾 Invert the urine sample to ensure that it is thoroughly mixed.
- 🐾 Dip the stick into the urine sample until all of the reagent pads are wet.
- 🐾 Quickly remove the stick and gently tap the stick on the side of the urine pot to remove excess urine.
- 🐾 Use the timer to ensure you keep to the correct time intervals as stated on the dipstick container's instructions.
- 🐾 Holding the correct end of the stick in one hand and the container in the other, compare the colour changes of each reagent pad with the side of the container.
- 🐾 Record your results on paper.

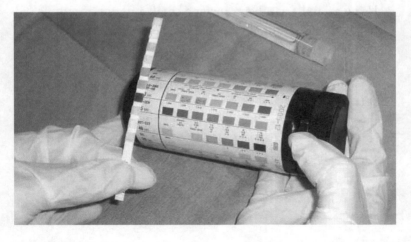

Figure 6.11 Urine and dipstick container and dipstick

LABORATORY TECHNIQUES

Case Study

6 Blood smear processing

You must be able to prepare a fresh blood smear correctly. Failure to do so could result in misdiagnosis of the patient's condition and a delay in the correct treatment. A fresh blood smear should be prepared for every haematology sample being sent to an external laboratory. Any defects in the blood smear must be noted and a possible explanation given as to what caused the defect as well as how to avoid it in subsequent blood smear tests.

Practical tips

Blood smear preparation

- Clean the slide with alcohol to degrease it.
- Invert the chosen sample to ensure it is thoroughly mixed.
- Put gloves on.
- Using a capillary tube, transfer a small amount of sample onto one end of the slide.
- Hold the slide spreader at a 30° angle to the microscope slide and draw it backwards until it touches the sample of blood.
- The blood will now spread along the edge of the slide spreader.
- Push the slide spreader along the microscope slide in a smooth and swift action.
- Air dry the smear.

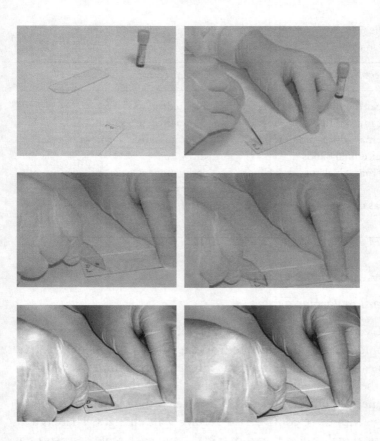

Figure 6.12 Blood smear preparation

Table 6.1 · Typical defects in blood smear preparation and common explanations

Defect	Explanation
Smear too thick or too long	Blood drop too large
Smear too thin or too short	Blood drop too small
Alternate thick and thin longitudinal bands	Contamination of spreader, usually dirt
Alternate thick and thin bands	Jerky movement of spreader, usually poor technique used, or nerves!
Areas of no blood or patchy blood	Insufficient cleaning of slide prior to use

Revision notes

Reading vernier scales

The vernier scale enables you to relocate the item on a slide should the slide be removed from the microscope. This will save time and effort if the item was difficult to find initially. Located on the stage are the direction controls, and the vernier scales are connected to these controls; whenever you move the slide on the stage with these controls, the vernier scale changes. There is a vertical scale and a horizontal scale, and each scale consists of a main scale with millimeter divisions and a smaller vernier scale reading from 0 to 10. The readings are very similar to map co-ordinates.

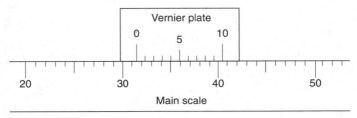

Figure 6.13 Vernier scale

1 The first part of the reading is taken from the main scale.
   The number opposite the 0 on the scale should be read;
   should it lie between two numbers, read the lowest number.
2 Look on the vernier plate to find out which line lies directly
   opposite a line on the main scale; record this reading.
3. Repeat this process for the other scale.

It doesn't matter whether you read the horizontal scale or the
vertical reading first, just ensure you give the main scale first
then the vernier scale.

Example:

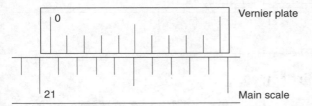

The zero is between 21 and 22 on the main scale. The line on
the vernier plate directly opposite a line on the main scale is at
number 6. This reading is therefore at 21.6.

Quick test

(Answers on page 144)

Have a practice at reading these vernier scales.

1

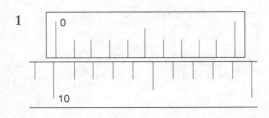

2

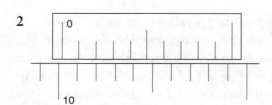

10.2

3

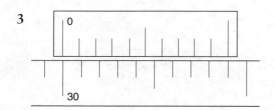

30.9

4

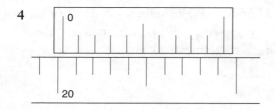

20.3

5

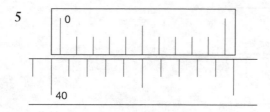

40.5

6

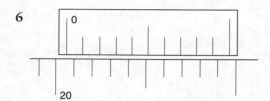

20·6

7

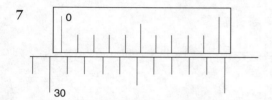

30·7

8

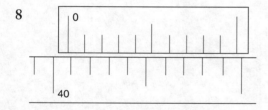

40·8

Chapter 7
Medical Nursing

Introduction

Medical nursing skills must always be performed in a safe and proficient manner. These nursing skills allow you to work closely with the patient – something which veterinary surgeons do not have time to do. Performing these nursing skills, and seeing the patient recover, is the main reason most people choose to become veterinary nurses; as such, it is vitally important that these skills are performed correctly. Using the correct nursing skills can be a very rewarding aspect of a VN's day-to-day work.

The VN plays an extremely important role in the recovery process and the aim of these skills is to help the patient return to a state of normal health as soon as possible. There are many skills encompassing medical nursing – the dispensing of drugs, performing physiotherapy, providing nutritional support, to name but a few – and it is important that they are carried out competently and proficiently to ensure the rapid recovery of any patient. The care you give must be based on a thorough understanding of the various disease processes and the aims of the treatment protocols.

What you need to know

Anatomy and physiology

- To be performed correctly, most medical nursing relies on a good knowledge of anatomy and physiology.
- Incorrect knowledge may harm your patient and slow down the recovery process.

Equipment and safe practice

- You must be able to identify and select equipment appropriately.
- You must be able to handle all equipment safely, with due respect for the patient, yourself, colleagues and clients.

Calculations and safe practice

- All calculations must be correctly performed.
- Even though the ultimate responsibility for ensuring that the correct drug dose is administered lies with the Veterinary Surgeon, you must be able to perform calculations correctly.
- Incorrect drug calculations can lead to patient deterioration or even death.
- Examples of drug dose calculations are given in the case studies below, and examples for you to practise are given at the end of the section.

Safe working environment

- Everyone has the right to work in a safe environment and you must know how to contribute to that safety within the area of nursing skills.

The following case studies are helpful illustrations of what to do in practice.

Case Study 1 — **Revival and resuscitation of neonates**

You are expected to know how to safely and correctly revive neonates following caesarean section. Failure to do so could result in death of the neonate. Any neonate is extremely fragile just after birth and as such a lot of irreparable damage can be done by using the incorrect technique. The following advice is for kittens as well as puppies.

Practical tips

NB 'Swinging' puppies has been found to cause head trauma and should not be performed.

Practical technique

- ☙ Put on an apron and gloves.
- ☙ Hold out a towel in both hands to allow the surgical assistant to 'drop' the puppy into the open towel – do not touch the surgical assistant.
- ☙ Rub the puppy vigorously with the towel to stimulate respiration, and almost immediately you have done this, check for a heartbeat.
- ☙ If there is no heartbeat, follow a resuscitation procedure of cardiac massage at a rate of approximately 200 beats per minute.
- ☙ This should be carried out using the finger and thumb of one hand whilst supporting the puppy with the other hand.
- ☙ Check for a heartbeat every 15 seconds.
- ☙ If there is a heartbeat, continue to rub the puppy vigorously with the towel to stimulate respiration.
- ☙ The puppy should start to show respiratory movement and the mucous membranes should be pink.

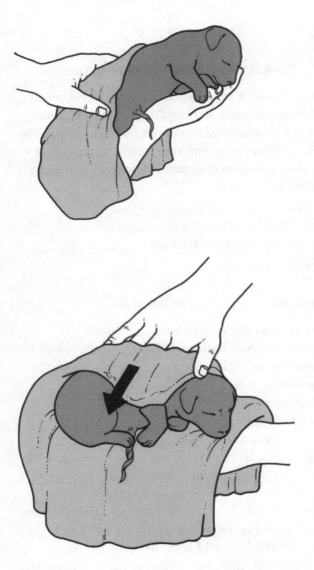

Figure 7.1   Neonate resuscitation

Case Study 2   Naso-oesophageal feeding

You must safely and correctly calculate the basal metabolic requirements for any inpatient, whether it is recovering from illness or as part of its illness treatment. Administering this food via a feeding tube is also an important nursing aspect as you could quite easily cause patient deterioration if it is not performed correctly.

For ease of explanation, the following text describes administering 20 ml of food, but in practice you may need to administer either more or less than this.

Practical tips

Calculation of daily dietary requirement

1 Work out the basal energy requirement (BER) first:
   - Small dogs and cats: BER = 60 kcal/kg × body weight (in kg) per 24 hours
   - Dogs over 5 kg: BER = (30 kcal/kg × (body weight in kg)) + 70 kcal per 24 hours.
2 Then multiply the BER by the disease factor; this will give you the daily energy requirement in kcal/24 hours.

Table 7.1

Condition	Disease Factor
Hospitalised dog / cat	1.3
Major trauma / surgery	1.6
Neoplasia	1.6
Severe infection or sepsis	1.8
Major burns	2.0

MEDICAL NURSING

3 Select the most suitable diet.
4 Divide the total energy requirement (in kcal) by the number of kcal/ml – this will give you the amount (in ml) to feed in 24 hours.
5 Divide this amount by the amount of feeds per day – this will give you the amount to feed per meal.

Feeding technique

* Put on an apron and gloves.
* Draw up 20 ml, for example, of the correct diet into a syringe.
* Draw up 2 × 5 ml of sterile saline into syringes.
* Attach one 5-ml syringe containing sterile saline onto the feeding tube and carefully push the syringe plunger.

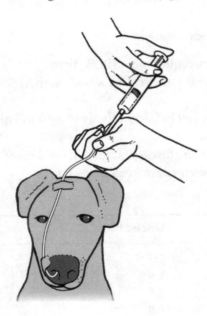

Figure 7.2 Feeding technique

- Disconnect the 5-ml syringe and attach the 20-ml syringe containing the liquid food.
- Slowly push the plunger until the syringe is empty.
- Disconnect the 20-ml syringe and attach the final 5-ml syringe of sterile saline.
- Carefully push the plunger until the syringe is empty.
- Remove the syringe and close the end of the feeding tube.

Case Study 3 — Calculating drug doses

You must safely and correctly dispense drugs to clients under the Veterinary Surgeon's instructions. Incorrect drug calculations can lead to patient deterioration or patient death should the wrong drug be dispensed or the wrong instructions be given to owners. It is the VN's responsibility to ensure drugs are dispensed correctly and safely and that the drug label conforms to legal requirements.

The following example is a useful way to illustrate what is involved in calculating drug doses.

Example: A canine patient belonging to Mrs Jones, 2 New St, Exeter is to be discharged with enough oxytetracycline tablets for a given number of weeks. (Veterinary Surgeon address Mr Smith MRCVS, 1 High Street, Exeter). The tablet size is given on the packaging and the dosage regime is written in the prescription.

How do we calculate the required dose and prepare the correct number of tablets needed?

Practical tips

Drug calculation

1 First work out the patient's daily dose:
   - Patient's weight (in kg) × dose rate (in mg/kg) = daily dose (in mg).
2 Divide this by the size of tablet available:
   - Daily dose (mg) ÷ tablet size (mg) = number of tablets per day.
3 Multiply this by the number of days for treatment:

- Number of tablets per day × number of days treatment
  = total amount of tablets for dispensing.
4 Divide the number of tablets per day by the number of doses per day:
  - Number of tablets per day ÷ number of doses per day
    = number of tablets per dose.

Practical technique

- Put gloves on.
- Select the correct tablet strength and check the expiry date.
- Count the required number of tablets.
- Place the tablets into the correct tablet container.
- Write a label according to correct legislation.
- Attach the label to the container.
- Ensure the container is secure.

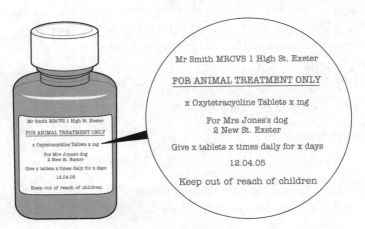

Figure 7.3 A tablet bottle and a drug label

Revision notes

Drug dosage calculations

Example: A 20-kg dog is to be discharged with enough 100-mg tablets for 2 weeks. The dose rate is 10 mg/kg per day in two equal doses. What is the dog's required dose and how many tablets should you dispense?

1 First we need to work out the patient's daily dose.
2 Multiply the patient's weight by the dose rate:
   • 20 kg × 10 mg/kg = 200 mg per day is required.
3 Then we need to divide this dose by the size of tablet available, in this case it is 100 mg:
   • 200 mg ÷ 100 mg = 2 tablets.
4 Multiply this by the number of days treatment, 2 weeks = 14 days:
   • 2 tablets × 14 days = 28 tablets.
5 The patient will need 28 tablets.
6 Divide the number of tablets per day by the number of doses per day:
   • 2 tablets ÷ 2 doses = 1.
7 So one tablet will be needed twice daily by the patient, and 28 tablets will be needed in total.

Quick test

(Answers on page 144)

Calculate the drug dosages for the following patients

1 A patient is to be discharged with enough tablets for
2 weeks. Calculate the required dose and the number of
tablets required:
  * tablet size 50 mg each
  * dog's weight is 25 kg
  * dose rate is 2 mg/kg per day in two equal doses.

½ tablet twice daily =14 tabs

2 A patient is to be discharged with enough tablets for
1 week. Calculate the required dose and the number of
tablets required:
  * tablet size 200 mg each
  * dog's weight is 10 kg
  * dose rate is 20 mg/kg per day in two equal doses.

½ tablet twice daily = 7 tabs

3 A patient is to be discharged with enough tablets for
3 weeks. Calculate the required dose and the number of
tablets required:
  * tablet size 20 mg each
  * dog's weight is 2 kg
  * dose rate is 40 mg/kg per day in four equal doses.

1 tab. four daily = 84 tabs.

4   A patient is to be discharged with enough tablets for
    1 week. Calculate the required dose and the number of
    tablets required:
    ❧ tablet size 250 mg each
    ❧ dog's weight is 30 kg
    ❧ dose rate is 25 mg/kg per day in two equal doses.

1 ½ tabs dwice daily = 21 tabs

5   A patient is to be discharged with enough tablets for
    2 weeks. Calculate the required dose and the number of
    tablets required:
    ❧ tablet size 80 mg each
    ❧ dog's weight is 8 kg
    ❧ dose rate is 10 mg/kg per day in two equal doses.

1/2 tab twice daily = 14 tabs

6   A patient is to be discharged with enough tablets for
    3 weeks. Calculate the required dose and the number of
    tablets required:
    ❧ tablet size 50 mg each
    ❧ dog's weight is 25 kg
    ❧ dose rate is 4 mg/kg per day in four equal doses.

1/2 tab four daily = 42 tabs

Case Study 4 **Urinary catheterisation**

You are expected to prepare equipment for urinary catheterisation, check that it is functional and check urinary output. You may be expected to nurse a urinary patient, therefore knowledge of these procedures and equipment required is vital.

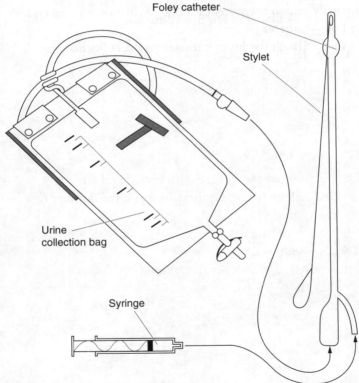

Foley catheter

Stylet

Urine collection bag

Syringe

Figure 7.4 Connected equipment

MEDICAL NURSING

Practical tips

Practical technique

* Check the amount of sterile water that can be placed within the balloon of the Foley catheter and draw this up into a syringe.
* Slowly inject the sterile water through the correct portion of the Foley catheter – the balloon should now increase in size – do not squeeze the balloon or this will pop with the pressure of water inside it!
* Correctly attach the stylet into one of the holes at the end of the Foley catheter.
* Correctly attach the Foley catheter to the collection bag.

Case Study 5 Physiotherapy

You must safely and correctly perform physiotherapy on any inpatient. Performing physiotherapy incorrectly can have detrimental results on your patient, not to mention causing considerable pain. Bladder expression can be very painful for the patient if it is not carried out correctly. Pressure sores should not be allowed to occur, therefore knowledge of areas of susceptibility is important.

Examples are given below to illustrate best physiotherapy practice.

Example: Positioning and coupage to minimise the possibility of hypostatic pneumonia developing.

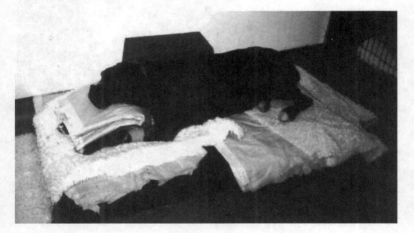

Figure 7.5   Patient in sternal recumbency

MEDICAL NURSING

Practical tips

🐾 Position the patient in sternal recumbency.
🐾 If necessary, use positioning aids to prevent the patient from falling over.

Coupage technique

🐾 With the patient still in sternal recumbency, gently percuss the thorax with cupped hands.
🐾 Starting at the caudal aspect of the thorax, work towards the cranial aspect.
🐾 Percuss both sides of the thorax.
🐾 This technique should encourage coughing and removal of secretions.

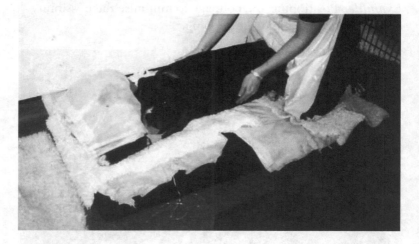

Figure 7.6   Coupage

Example: Bladder expression to relieve retention.

Practical tips

Bladder expression technique

- ❀ Ask an assistant to restrain the patient in a safe and appropriate manner.
- ❀ Place one hand on either side of the caudal abdominal wall.
- ❀ Isolate the bladder by palpating the caudal abdomen.
- ❀ Gently apply pressure to either side of the abdominal wall to squeeze the bladder.
- ❀ If there is resistance and no urine flow, stop the procedure.

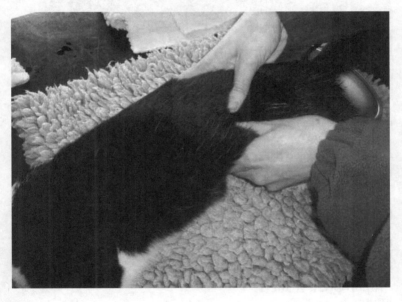

Figure 7.7   Bladder expression

MEDICAL NURSING

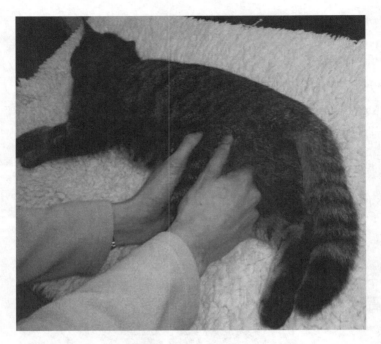

Figure 7.8   Patient receiving physiotherapy

Example: Physiotherapy for the hind limbs of a cat to minimise the risks of developing pressure sores.

Practical tips

Physiotherapy technique

- Ensure the patient is restrained by an assistant in a safe and appropriate manner.
- Perform effleurage on the cat's hind limbs; this is done by stroking the limbs in the direction of venous return.
- Perform petrissage on the cat's hind limbs; this is done by kneading the limbs in the direction of venous return.
- Perform friction on the cat's hind limbs; this is done by briskly rubbing the limbs in the direction of venous return.

Case Study 6

Diabetes mellitus management

You are expected to be able to work out the basal energy requirements for any patient and must also be able to select diets for any illness. Insulin is very easily destroyed by improper administration and usage and so using the correct technique for insulin storage, use and administration is very important.

Practical tips

Practical technique for giving insulin

- Select the appropriate size syringe and needle.
- Roll insulin bottle between hands gently.
- Remove required volume of drug from bottle.
- Remove any air bubbles in a safe manner.
- Replace cap before placing syringe on bench.

Injection technique

- Ensure the patient is restrained in a safe and appropriate manner.
- Raise a fold of skin to form a triangle.
- Insert the needle into the base of the triangle.
- Withdraw the plunger slightly to check it is not in a blood vessel.
- Inject drug if no blood appears in the syringe.
- Remove needle and massage area.
- Dispose of needle and syringe safely.

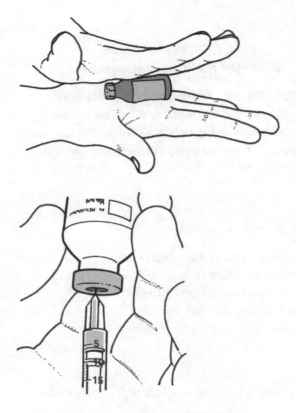

Figure 7.9   Bottle rolling and drawing up of drug

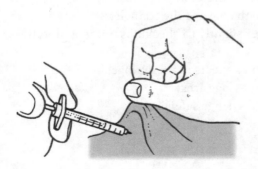

Figure 7.10   Injection technique

Revision notes

Basal energy requirement (BER) calculations

Use the following formulae to work out the BER:

🐾 For small dogs and cats (under 5 kg): use formula (a):
   BER = 60 kcal/kg × (body weight in kg) kcal/24 hours
🐾 For larger dogs (over 5 kg): use formula (b):
   BER = (30 kcal/kg × (body weight in kg)) + 70 kcal/24 hours.

Example: An adult dog weighing 10 kg needs 2 times its basal energy requirement. Calculate the daily energy requirements for this patient. How much food would you give per day if six daily feeds were given?

1 This dog weighs 10 kg, so the correct formula to use would be (b).
2 Substitute the body weight in the correct area of the formula:
   • BER = (30 kcal/kg × 10 kg) + 70 kcal.
3 Carry out the first part of the formula first, ie 30 kcal/kg × 10 kg, then add the 70 kcal:
   • BER = 300 + 70 kcal.
4 So the BER for this patient would be 370 kcal/24 hours.
5 But, this dog needs twice its BER; therefore, we multiply his BER by 2
   • 2 × 370 = 740 kcal/24 hours.
6 To go further, we need to know the calorie density of the food.
7 Use the following formula:
   • Volume to feed = (total requirement in kcal/day) ÷ (energy density of chosen food in kcal/ml).
8 So, let's assume the calorie density of the food is 1.2 kcal/ml.
9 We need to divide the patient's required energy (in kcal/day) by the energy density (in kcal per ml) of food:
   740 kcal/day ÷ 1.2 kcal/ml = 617 ml/day of diet.

10 So the patient requires 617 ml of diet per 24 hours.

11 We then need to divide it by the number of meals per day, which is six:

617 ml ÷ 6 = 103 ml per feed.

12 So this patient would need 103 ml of food per meal.

Quick test

(Answers on page 144)

Calculate the daily energy requirements for the following patients

1 An adult dog weighing 20 kg requires 1.5 times its basal energy requirement. How much food would you give per day if four daily feeds were given? Assume the chosen food to be 4 kcal/ml. How much food would you give per meal?

. .25ml per day , 63ml .feed

2 An adult dog weighing 33 kg requires 1.3 times its basal energy requirement. How much food would you give per day if six daily feeds were given? Assume the chosen food to be 2 kcal/ml. How much food would you give per meal?

.689 ml per. day., 115ml feed

3 An adult dog weighing 8 kg requires 1.7 times its basal energy requirement. How much food would you give per day if six daily feeds were given? Assume the chosen food to be 6 kcal/ml. How much food would you give per meal?

88ml perday., 15ml. feed . . .

4 An adult dog weighing 25 kg requires 1.3 times its basal energy requirement. How much food would you give per day if nine daily feeds were given? Assume the chosen food to be 4 kcal/ml. How much food would you give per meal?

. 266 ml per day, 30ml feed

5 An adult dog weighing 20 kg requires 1.7 times its basal energy requirement. How much food would you give per day if nine daily feeds were given? Assume the chosen food to be 1.5 kcal/ml. How much food would you give per meal?

. 759 ml per day. 84 ml feed

6 An adult dog weighing 12 kg requires two times its basal energy requirement. How much food would you give per day if six daily feeds were given? Assume the chosen food to be 2 kcal/ml. How much food would you give per meal?

. 430 ml per day., 72ml feed

7 An adult dog weighing 18 kg requires 1.5 times its basal energy requirement. How much food would you give per day if four daily feeds were given? Assume the chosen food to be 5 kcal/ml. How much food would you give per meal?

. 183ml per day. 46ml feed

8 An adult dog weighing 30 kg requires two times its basal energy requirement. How much food would you give per day if nine daily feeds were given? Assume the chosen food to be 1.6 kcal/ml. How much food would you give per meal?

1212ml per day, 135ml feed

9 An adult dog weighing 4 kg requires two times its basal energy requirement. How much food would you give per day if six daily feeds were given? Assume the chosen food to be 6 kcal/ml. How much food would you give per meal?

80ml per day, 13ml feed.

10 An adult dog weighing 17 kg requires 1.7 times its basal energy requirement. How much food would you give per day if six daily feeds were given? Assume the chosen food to be 2 kcal/ml. How much food would you give per meal?

493ml per day 82ml feed

11 An adult dog weighing 27 kg requires 1.3 times its basal energy requirement. How much food would you give per day if nine daily feeds were given? Assume the chosen food to be 1.2 kcal/ml. How much food would you give per meal?

953ml per day, 106ml.

12 An adult dog weighing 38 kg requires two times its basal
    energy requirement. How much food would you give per
    day if nine daily feeds were given? Assume the chosen food
    to be 2 kcal/ml. How much food would you give per meal?

.1210 ml per day, 134ml feed

13 An adult dog weighing 12 kg requires 1.3 times its basal
    energy requirement. How much food would you give per
    day if four daily feeds were given? Assume the chosen food
    to be 4 kcal/ml. How much food would you give per meal?

. 140 ml per day., 35ml feed

Chapter 8
Radiography

Introduction

The production of radiographs can be very rewarding for a VN. As such, it is very important that you are able to position an animal to produce a diagnostic radiograph. To achieve consistently good radiographs is invaluable and, to accomplish this, a standardised positioning technique is employed together with standard centring points and collimation areas.

What you need to know

Radiographic positioning

* You must be able to position the patient for each and every exposure to be made.
* Inadequate positioning will necessitate a repeat of exposures which is against the Ionising Radiations Regulations (1999).
* Ensure you know the results of your exposure before you say you will press the exposure button!
* Before you begin, ensure your cassette is within the primary beam and is collimated to the edges of the cassette.

Equipment and safe practice

* Whenever a patient is positioned for radiography, consideration should be given as to why the animal is being radiographed.

❧ Care should be taken to avoid worsening any condition that the patient may be suffering from.

❧ A good knowledge of anatomy will be invaluable in the positioning of your patients for radiography.

Anatomical landmarks

❧ For every position, there are distinct landmarks which should be used to ensure that you have centred the beam appropriately over the correct area.

Safe practice

❧ Radiography can be dangerous if used inappropriately: the beam should be centred correctly over the area to be exposed and it should also be collimated to reduce the effect of scattered radiation.

❧ Knowledge of the collimation areas is also necessary.

❧ Animals must not be held for radiography under any circumstance.

❧ Positioning aids are used during veterinary radiography to ensure that limbs and other body parts do not infiltrate the exposure area, as this would obliterate your film.

❧ However, these positioning aids can be used detrimentally with inadequate knowledge.

❧ Write your patient's details (include the date) on the x-rite tape and have your L/R marker handy. Use a grid if the area you are x-raying is more than 10 cm deep.

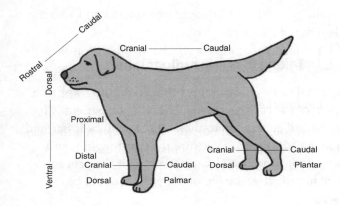

Figure 8.1 Anatomical directions for radiography

The following case studies are helpful illustrations of what to do in practice.

Case Study

Taking thoracic radiographs

You are expected to be able to take a thoracic radiograph of a conscious patient for various reasons. Maybe the patient is too ill to be given a full general anaesthetic (GA). Maybe it has had a road accident and we need to ensure the diaphragm is still intact before administering a GA. Either way, if the procedure is undertaken incorrectly, the life of the patient could be compromised.

Practical tips

Positioning technique for a lateral thoracic radiograph

- Position your patient in right lateral recumbency ensuring the thorax is over the cassette.
- Your patient is conscious, so ensure you do not handle them too roughly.
- Extend the patient's head and place a sandbag over the neck to ensure they can't sit up during the exposure.
- Extend the front legs cranially and secure in place.
- Extend the hind legs caudally and secure in place.
- Place a foam wedge underneath the sternum to prevent rotation of the patient.
- Check to ensure your patient is straight and not rotated.
- Ensure none of your sandbags are in the primary beam.
- Ensure the patient's identification and that the R marker is visible within the collimated area.

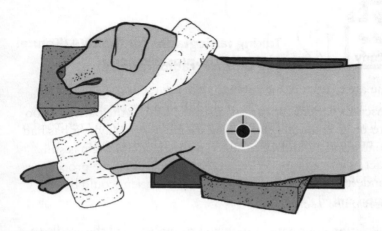

Figure 8.2   Lateral thorax positioning

Table 8.1   Guide to correct positioning for radiography

Centre the beam	At the caudal border of the scapula, midway between the dorsal scapula and sternum
Dorsal collimation	Include the dorsal border of the scapula
Ventral collimation	Include the ventral border of the sternum
Cranial collimation	Include the thoracic inlet/manubrium
Caudal collimation	Include the last rib

RADIOGRAPHY

Case Study 2

Taking radiographs for the BVA/Kennel Club Hip Dysplasia scheme

You are expected to be able to take a radiograph suitable for submission to the BVA/Kennel Club Hip Dysplasia scheme. Failure to do so will result in your radiograph being returned to the practice and the necessity to repeat the exposure.

Practical tips

Positioning technique

- 🐾 Position your patient in dorsal recumbency in the cradle to prevent rotation.
- 🐾 Ensure the cradle is not over the cassette otherwise this would show up on your radiograph.
- 🐾 Extend both hind limbs and secure with ties placed around the 'hocks' and secure to the table (the table may have cleats for you to attach ties to, but if not, secure with a sandbag).
- 🐾 Rotate the limbs medially and secure in place with tape (ask your assistant to hold the limbs in place while you secure with tape).
- 🐾 Place an additional sandbag over the hind feet to bring the area closer to the cassette.
- 🐾 Check to ensure the patient's body isn't rotated.
- 🐾 Check the patient's Kennel Club number and date and that the R/L marker is placed correctly and is visible within the collimated area.

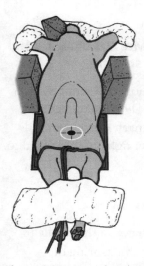

Figure 8.3 Ventrodorsal pelvis

Table 8.2 Guide to correct positioning for radiography

Centre the beam	Level with the cranial border of the pubic symphysis or the cranial border of the greater trochanters
Lateral collimation	Level with lateral skin surfaces of the pelvis
Cranial collimation	Include iliac wings
Caudal collimation	Include the midshaft of the femurs

RADIOGRAPHY

Case Study 3

Taking a lateral survey radiograph of the spine

You are expected to be able to take a lateral survey radiograph of the spine. The spine must be totally straight and parallel to the cassette. Due to divergence of the primary x-ray beam, failure to ensure that the spine is totally straight could to lead to misdiagnosis of the patient's condition.

Practical tips

Positioning technique

- Position the patient in lateral recumbency ensuring the cervical spine is on the cassette.
- Place foam wedges under the sternum, nose and between the front limbs to ensure no rotation occurs.
- Add additional small foam wedges under the cervical spine to ensure the spine is totally straight with no sagging.
- Extend the front limbs caudally and secure in place.
- Extend the hind limbs caudally and secure in place.
- Check to ensure the patient's body is totally straight.
- Ensure the patient's identification and R/L marker are visible within the collimated area.

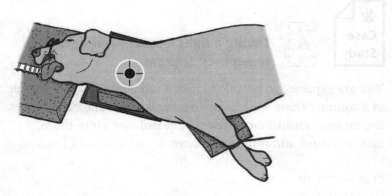

Figure 8.4   Lateral cervical spine

Table 8.3   Guide to correct positioning for radiography

Centre the beam	Level with C4
Dorsal collimation	Include the dorsal skin border
Ventral collimation	Include the ventral skin border
Cranial collimation	Include the occipital process
Caudal collimation	Include the caudal border of the scapula

RADIOGRAPHY

Case Study

Taking a right lateral pneumocystogram

You are expected to be able to take a radiograph of the bladder as a contrast study. Failure to do so will incur repeat exposures and an increase in anaesthetic time. Misdiagnosis of the patient's condition could also occur.

Practical tips

Administering contrast for pneumocystogram

- ❀ Aseptically place a urinary catheter into the patient's urethra.
- ❀ Remove any urine from the patient's bladder.
- ❀ Attach a 3-way tap to the end of the catheter.
- ❀ Using a syringe, instill air into the bladder until the bladder is palpable.
- ❀ Ensure air cannot leak out of the 3-way tap or catheter.

Positioning technique

- ❀ Position the patient in right lateral recumbency ensuring the abdomen is over the cassette.
- ❀ Extend the forelimbs and secure in place.
- ❀ Extend the hind limbs and secure in place.
- ❀ Place a foam wedge underneath the sternum to prevent rotation of the patient.
- ❀ Check to ensure the patient's body isn't rotated.
- ❀ Ensure the patient identification and that the R marker is visible within the collimated area.

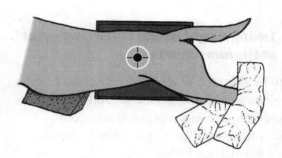

Figure 8.5 Lateral abdomen and bladder

Table 8.4 Guide to correct placement for radiography

Centre the beam	Cranial to the wing of the ileum midway between the skin edges of the spine and abdomen
Dorsal collimation	Include the skin edges of the abdomen
Ventral collimation	Include the skin edges of the lumbar-sacral spine
Cranial collimation	Include the last rib
Caudal collimation	Include the skin edges of the ischium

RADIOGRAPHY

Case Study

5 Taking a right lateral survey radiograph of the lumbar spine

You are expected to be able to take a lateral survey radiograph of the spine. The spine must be totally straight and parallel to the cassette. Due to divergence of the primary x-ray beam, failure to ensure the spine is totally straight could to lead to misdiagnosis of the patient's condition.

Practical tips

Positioning technique

- Position the patient in lateral recumbency ensuring the lumbar spine is on the cassette.
- Place foam wedges under the thorax, nose, between the stifles and the front limbs.
- Add additional padding under the cervical and lumbar spine to ensure the spine is totally straight with no rotation.
- Secure the front limbs and hind limbs with a sandbag, ensuring they are in extension.
- Check to ensure the patient's body isn't rotated.
- Ensure the patient identification and that the R marker is visible within the collimated area.

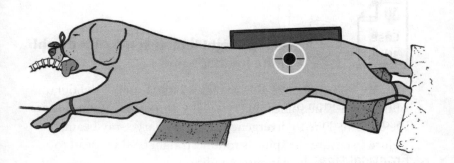

Figure 8.6   Lateral lumbar spine positioning

Table 8.5   Guide to correct positioning for radiography

Centre the beam	Midway between thoracolumbar junction and iliac crest, at L4
Dorsal collimation	Include dorsal skin surface of spine
Ventral collimation	Include the mid abdomen
Cranial collimation	Include thoracolumbar junction
Caudal collimation	Include iliac crest

RADIOGRAPHY

Case Study

Taking a lateral radiograph of the right tibia

You are expected to be able to take a radiograph of the tibia. Limb dislocation or fractures could occur if positioning aids are used incorrectly.

Practical tips

Positioning technique

- Position the patient in right lateral recumbency.
- Ensure the right tibia is over the cassette.
- Secure the left leg out of the way using a tie.
- Pull the fore limbs cranially and secure in position.
- Secure the right limb in position.
- A foam wedge may be necessary, either under the stifle or the hock, to ensure the tibia is parallel to the cassette.
- Ensure the patient's identification and that the R marker is visible within the collimated area.

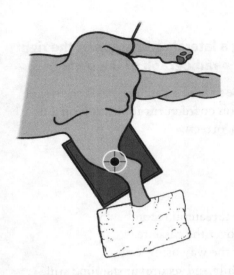

Figure 8.7   Lateral right tibia positioning

Table 8.6   Guide to correct positioning for radiography

Centre the beam	Mid-shaft of the tibia
Dorsal collimation	Include the distal third of the femur
Ventral collimation	Include the tarsal joint
Cranial and caudal collimation	Include the skin edges of the limb

RADIOGRAPHY

Case Study 7

Taking a radiograph of the stifle

You are expected to be able to take a caudocranial radiograph of the stifle. Limb dislocation or fractures could occur if positioning aids are used incorrectly.

Practical tips

Positioning technique

- Place the patient in sternal recumbency.
- Extend the limbs caudally.
- Secure the front limbs.
- Elevate the left stifle with sandbags so that the right stifle is straight.
- Secure the right limb in position.
- Ensure the patient's identification and that the R marker is visible within the collimated area.

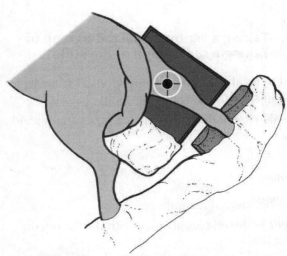

Figure 8.8   Caudocranial stifle positioning

Table 8.7   Guide to correct positioning for radiography

Centre the beam	Through the stifle joint
Dorsal collimation	Include the distal third of the femur
Ventral collimation	Include the proximal third of the tibia
Cranial and caudal collimation	Include the skin edges of the stifle

RADIOGRAPHY

Case Study 8

Taking a ventrodorsal radiograph of the thorax

You are expected to be able to take a ventrodorsal radiograph of the thorax correctly. Placing the patient in the wrong position could be detrimental, as could placing positioning aids incorrectly.

Practical tips

Positioning technique

- Place the patient in dorsal recumbency with the thorax on the cassette.
- If you are using a trough for support, ensure you can still see all of your cassette.
- Extend the fore limbs cranially and secure in place.
- Extend the hind limbs caudally and secure in place.
- Ensure the patient is not rotated.
- Ensure the patient's identification and that the R/L marker is visible within the collimated area.

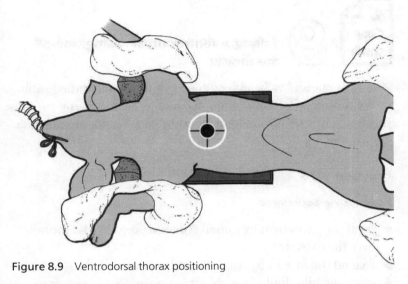

Figure 8.9 Ventrodorsal thorax positioning

Table 8.8 Guide to correct positioning for radiography

Centre the beam	To the midline, halfway along the sternum
Dorsal and ventral collimation	Include the skin edges of the thorax
Cranial collimation	Include the manubrium
Caudal collimation	Include the last rib

RADIOGRAPHY

Case Study 9

Taking a dorsoventral radiograph of the thorax

You are expected to be able to take a dorsoventral radiograph of the thorax correctly. Placing the patient in the wrong position could be detrimental, as could placing positioning aids incorrectly.

Practical tips

Positioning technique

- ☙ Position the patient in sternal recumbency with the thorax over the cassette.
- ☙ Extend the forelimbs cranially and secure in place.
- ☙ Place the hind limbs in a crouching position and secure in position with sandbags.
- ☙ Place a sandbag over the patient's neck but not as to compromise breathing.
- ☙ Place a foam wedge underneath the patient's chin.
- ☙ Ensure there is no patient rotation.
- ☙ Ensure the patient's identification and that the R/L marker is visible within the collimated area.

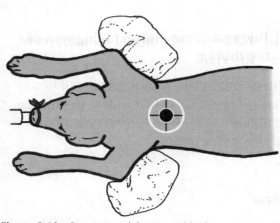

Figure 8.10   Dorsoventral thorax positioning

Table 8.9   Guide to correct positioning for radiography.

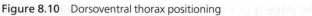

Centre the beam	To the midline, level with the caudal border of the scapula
Dorsal and ventral collimation	Include the skin edges of the thorax
Cranial collimation	Include the manubrium
Caudal collimation	Include the last rib

RADIOGRAPHY

Case Study 10
Taking a right lateral radiograph of the skull

You are expected to be able to take a skull radiograph correctly. The patient must not be rotated and the positioning aids used must not obliterate the area of interest, otherwise repeat exposures will be necessary.

Practical tips

Positioning technique

* Position the patient in right lateral recumbency with the skull on the cassette.
* Secure the front limbs in position.
* Place a foam wedge underneath the neck to prevent sagging.
* Place a foam wedge underneath the nose and mandible to ensure the interpupillary line is perpendicular to the cassette.
* A tie may be necessary, placed across the patient's muzzle to bring it closer to the cassette.
* Ensure the patient's identification and that the R marker is visible within the collimated area.

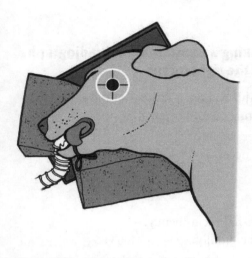

Figure 8.11   Right lateral skull positioning

Table 8.10   Guide to correct positioning for radiography

Centre the beam	Half way between the eye and the ear
Dorsal collimation	Include the skin edges of the skull
Ventral collimation	Include the skin edges of the mandible
Cranial collimation	Include the nostrils
Caudal collimation	Include the occipital process

RADIOGRAPHY

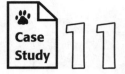

Taking a plantarodorsal radiograph of the right tarsus

You are expected to be able to take a radiograph of the tarsus. Limb dislocation or fractures could occur if positioning aids are used incorrectly.

Practical tips

Positioning technique

- Place the patient in sternal recumbency.
- Extend the hind limbs caudally.
- Secure the front limbs.
- Elevate the left stifle with sandbags so that the right tarsus is straight.
- Secure the right limb in position.
- Ensure the patient's identification and that the R marker is visible within the collimated area.

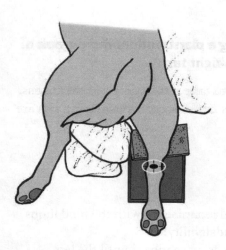

Figure 8.12   Plantarodorsal tarsus positioning

Table 8.11   Guide to correct positioning for radiography

Centre the beam	Through the mid-tarsal joint
Dorsal collimation	Include the distal third of the tibia
Ventral collimation	Include the mid-shaft metatarsals
Cranial and caudal collimation	Include the skin surfaces of the tarsus

RADIOGRAPHY

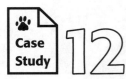

Case Study 12

Taking a dorsopalmar radiograph of the left carpus

You are expected to be able to take a radiograph of the carpus. Limb dislocation or fractures could occur if positioning aids are used incorrectly.

Practical tips

Positioning technique

- Place the patient in sternal recumbency with the hind limbs abducted to ensure patient stability.
- Elevate the right forelimb using sandbags until the left forelimb is straight.
- Extend the right fore limb cranially and secure in position.
- Ensure the patient's identification and that the L marker is visible within the collimated area.

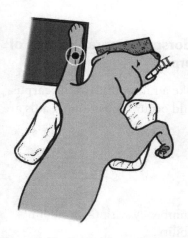

Figure 8.13 Dorsopalmar carpus positioning

Table 8.12 Guide to correct positioning for radiography

Centre the beam	Through the carpus
Dorsal and ventral collimation	Include the carpal skin edges
Caudal collimation	Include the toes
Cranial collimation	Include the mid-shaft radius/ulna

RADIOGRAPHY

Chapter 9
Surgical Nursing

Introduction

Theatre nursing and surgical nursing are all important areas of a VN's day-to-day work. It is usually the responsibility of the VN to organise all matters concerning the efficient running of the theatre within veterinary practice. The main focus of this area is to maintain aseptic technique and this is applied to all areas of theatre nursing, including instrument care and personal theatre hygiene.

The strict theatre protocols in place today are as a direct result of operating theatre personnel realising that an aseptic technique is required to help prevent post-operative infection. It is a myth that animals are more resistant to infection than humans and the standard operating theatre wear today should include gowns, gloves, hats and masks, etc. Instruments should also be sterilised correctly between each patient to prevent the transference of illness and disease.

What you need to know

Instruments

* You must be able to identify either general or orthopaedic instruments.
* As a nurse you will be involved in the care and maintenance

127

of surgical instruments and/or you will be a valuable member of the surgical team.

🐾 Knowledge of instrument names and uses will be invaluable when performing these tasks.

🐾 Schedule 3 legislation enables qualified and listed VNs to be able to suture wounds, so being able to hold instruments correctly will ensure the procedure is undertaken with the maximum of efficiency.

Suture materials

🐾 You must be able to identify the properties of suture material and have a sound knowledge of which materials are synthetic and which are natural.

🐾 There is a vast amount of suture materials available to the veterinary profession and new materials are constantly being produced.

Safe practical technique

🐾 You must correctly and safely don theatre clothing without breaking sterility.

🐾 Should sterility be broken, you must be able to recognise this and respond accordingly, as this could lead to infection gaining access to the surgical site and contamination of the surgical field.

🐾 Wound breakdown can occur when sterility is broken leading to infection and delayed wound healing.

🐾 You must be able to drape a trolley top in a sterile manner using Cheatle forceps.

The following case studies help to illustrate how you should carry out various surgical nursing in practice.

Case Study 1

Sterile gowning and gloving

You must be proficient at gowning and gloving and understand when sterility may be broken. VNs may be expected to glove and gown at a moment's notice and must be able to perform it competently and efficiently.

Practical tips

Gown donning procedure

* Pick up the inside of the gown at the shoulders.
* Move away from any surface and allow the gown to unfold gently without letting it touch the floor.
* Ensuring you touch only the inside of the gown, slide each arm into the sleeves.
* Ask an assistant to stand behind you and pull the gown so it fits over the shoulders (only by touching the gown inside).
* If you are going to close glove, ensure you keep your hands inside the cuffs at all times; however, if you are going to open glove, then your hands can come out of the cuffs.
* Ask an assistant to tie the ties at the back.
* Lean forwards so the front ties hang forwards (but not touching the floor).
* Grasp these front ties and hold them out so that the assistant can grasp the ends and tie them at the back of the gown.

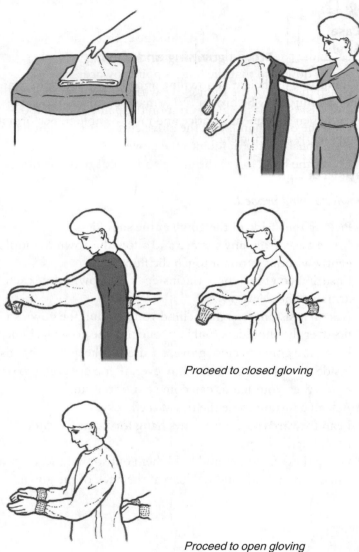

Proceed to closed gloving

Proceed to open gloving

Figure 9.1 Gown donning

Closed gloving

- 🐾 Ensure the hands are well within the cuffs of the gown.
- 🐾 Open the packet on the sterile field and turn the packet upside down, so that the fingers point towards you.
- 🐾 Grasp the cuff of the right glove with the right hand and turn the wrist over so the gloves rest on the palm of the hand.
- 🐾 With the other hand, pull the glove cuff over the right hand whilst pushing the hand into the glove.
- 🐾 Adjust the hand inside the glove and repeat with the other hand.

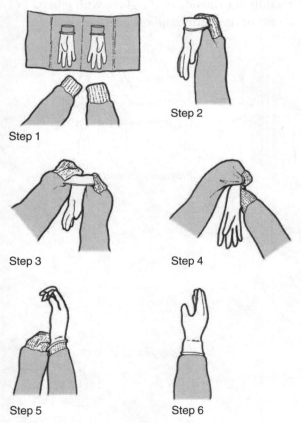

Step 1

Step 2

Step 3

Step 4

Step 5

Step 6

Figure 9.2   Closed gloving

Open gloving

- 🐾 Handle only the inside of the glove with ungloved hands.
- 🐾 Pick up the right glove with your left hand.
- 🐾 Pull the glove onto your right hand, ensuring the cuff becomes hooked over the right thumb.
- 🐾 Place the gloved right fingers under the cuff of the left glove and pull onto your left hand, only touching the outside of the glove.
- 🐾 Pull the cuff of the left glove over the cuff of the gown using the fingers of your right hand.
- 🐾 Again, touching only the outside of the glove with gloved hands, pull the cuff of the right hand over the cuff of the gown.

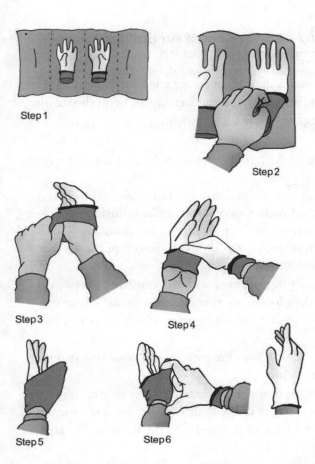

Step 1

Step 2

Step 3

Step 4

Step 5

Step 6

Figure 9.3   Open gloving

SURGICAL NURSING

Case Study 2 Preparation of surgical instrument trolley

You must be proficient at laying out a sterile trolley using Cheatle forceps without breaking sterility and you should also be able to recognise specific instruments.

Practical tips

Draping procedure

* Gently lift the Cheatle forceps out of the jar using their handles, ensuring you keep the tips lower than your hands.
* Using both forceps, gently lift the drape out of the 'sterile' container without touching the sides.
* Locate a corner of the drape with the Cheatle forceps in your right hand, then locate another corner with the Cheatle forceps in your left hand – be very careful not to drop the drape!
* Open out the drape with the forceps and walk towards the trolley to be draped.
* Gently place the drape over the trolley, being careful not to touch any part of the drape with your body – it is easier to drape from the back of the trolley to the front as you are less likely to break sterility.
* Let go of the drape carefully and replace the forceps back into the jar without touching the sides.

Instrument selection

* Select your instruments carefully and ensure you place them in the order required by the surgeon.

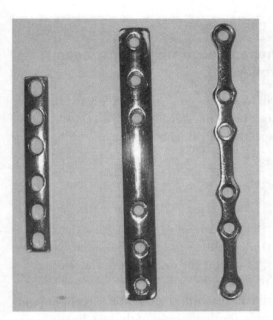

Figure 9.4   Bone plates: Dynamic compression plate, Venables plate and
Sherman plate

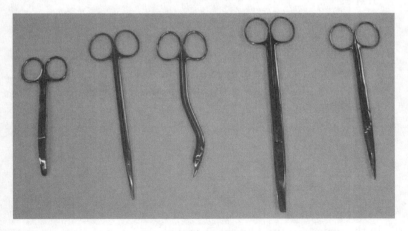

Figure 9.5   Scissors: dressing, Metzenbaum, Heath, Mayo and Mayo fine
tipped straight

SURGICAL NURSING

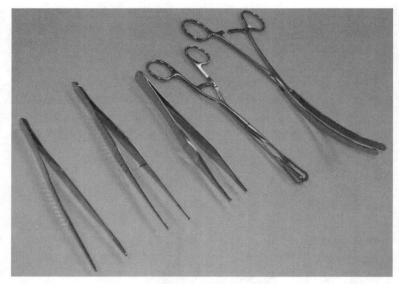

Figure 9.6 Forceps: plain dressing, Treves, Lane, Rampley's sponge-holding forceps and Doyen bowel clamp

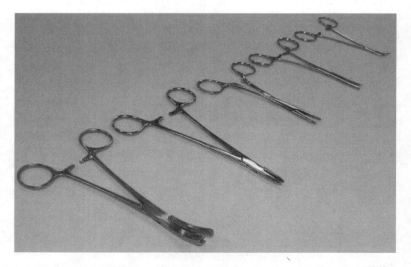

Figure 9.7 Ferguson angiotribes haemostat, Mayo needle holders, Spencer Wells forceps, Kocher and Halstead mosquito

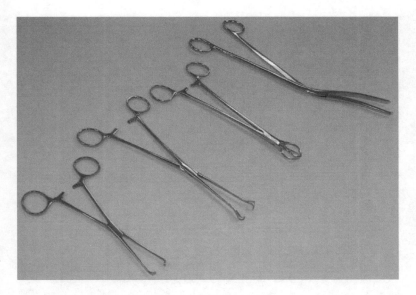

Figure 9.8   Forceps: Allis tissue, Babcock's tissue, Lane tissue and Cheatle forceps

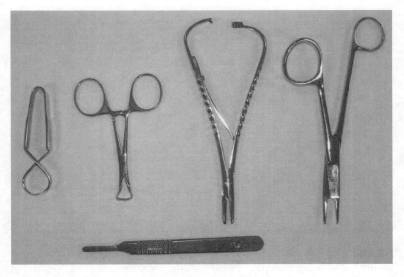

Figure 9.9   Cross-action towel clip, Backhaus towel clip, MacPhail's needle holders, Gilles needle holders and Bard-Parker scalpel handle

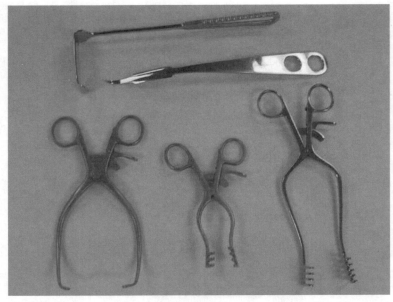

Figure 9.10   Retractors: Lagenbeck, Hohmann, Gelpi, West and Travers

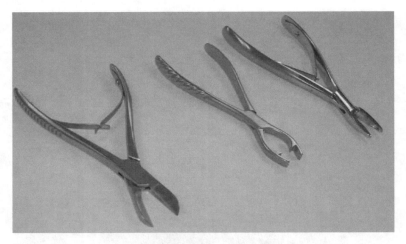

Figure 9.11   Liston bone cutters, Fergusson's bone-holding forceps and Lempert rongeurs

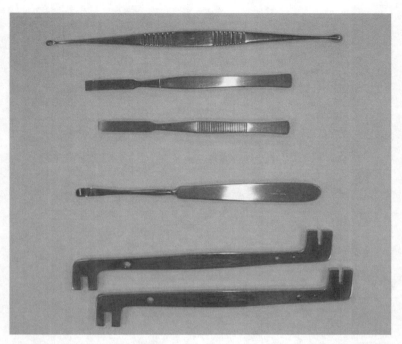

Figure 9.12 Volkman's scoop, chisel, osteotome, periosteal elevator and plate benders

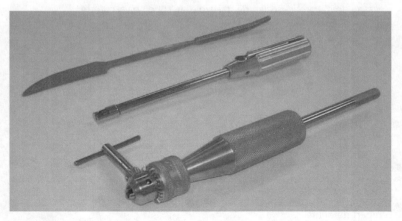

Figure 9.13 Rasp, orthopaedic screwdriver and Jacob's chuck

SURGICAL NURSING

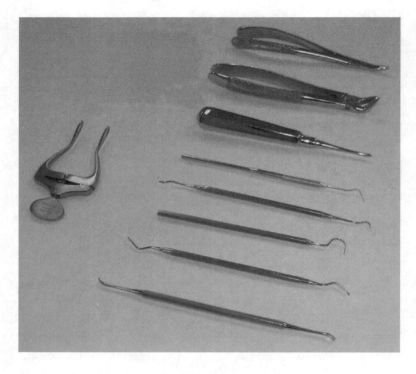

Figure 9.14 Left: rodent mouth gag. Right: dental extraction forceps, root elevator, dental probe, scaler, dental explorer, subgingival curette, double-ended dental scaler

Case Study **3** **Instrument recognition and handling**

You should be proficient at recognising and naming surgical instruments. Schedule 3 legislation enables qualified and listed VNs to be able to suture wounds, and being able to hold instruments correctly will ensure that the procedure is undertaken with the maximum of efficiency.

Commonly encountered sutures are of the following types:

* A synthetic absorbable monofilament suture
* A synthetic absorbable multifilament suture
* A synthetic non-absorbable monofilament suture
* A synthetic non-absorbable multifilament suture.

Practical tips

Instrument selection

* Select your instruments carefully and ensure you place them in the order required by the surgeon.

Instrument handling

* The correct way to hold scissors is by inserting the thumb and third index finger through the finger holes and resting the first index finger along the instrument shaft.
* This adds stability to the instrument whilst in use.

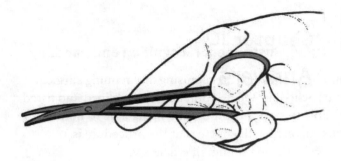

Figure 9.15 Scissor handling technique

🐾 The correct way to hold forceps is by holding them between your thumbs and index finger, just like you would do with a pen.

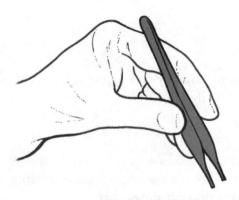

Figure 9.16 Forceps handling technique

Chapter 10
Answers

Anaesthetic Calculation Answers

1 3–3.8 litres
2 2.025–3.038 litres
3 3.9–4.7 litres
4 4.5–5.4 litres
5 14–16.8 litres
6 1.6–1.9 litres
7 3–3.6 litres
8 4.8–7.2 litres
9 5.6–8.4 litres
10 1.8–2.2 litres
11 2.7–4.05 litres
12 11–13.2 litres
13 5.3–7.9 litres
14 3.2–4.8 litres

Fluid Therapy Calculation Answers

1 175ml per day at a rate of 15 drops per minute
2 0.6 ml per minute which equals 8 drops per minute
3 1250 ml per day at a rate of 17 drops per minute
4 125 ml per day at a rate of 10 drops per minute
5 0.7 ml per minute which equals 10 drops per minute
6 600 ml per day at a rate of 17 drops per minute
7 135 ml per day at a rate of 11 drops per minute

8 0.5 ml per minute which equals 7 drops per minute
9 400 ml per day at a rate of 6 drops per minute
10 250 ml per day at a rate of 21 drops per minute
11 0.35 ml which equals a rate of 5 drops per minute
12 1750 ml per day at a rate of 24 drops per minute
13 100 ml per day at a rate of 4 drops per minute

Vernier Scale Answers

1 10.1
2 10.2
3 30.9
4 20.3
5 40.5
6 20.6
7 30.7
8 40.8

Drug Dosage Calculation Answers

1 Give $^1/_2$ a tablet twice daily = 14 tablets
2 Give $^1/_2$ a tablet twice daily = 7 tablets
3 Give 1 tablet 4 times daily = 84 tablets
4 Give $1^1/_2$ tablets twice daily = 21 tablets
5 Give $^1/_2$ a tablet twice daily = 14 tablets
6 Give $^1/_2$ tablet four times daily = 42 tablets

Daily Energy Requirement Calculation Answers

1 251 ml per day, 63 ml per feed
2 689 ml per day, 115 ml per feed
3 88 ml per day, 15 ml per feed
4 266 ml per day, 30 ml per feed
5 759 ml per day, 84 ml per feed
6 430 ml per day, 72 ml per feed

7 183 ml per day, 46 ml per feed
8 1212 ml per day, 135 ml per feed
9 80 ml per day, 13 ml per feed
10 493 ml per day, 82 ml per feed
11 953 ml per day, 106 ml per feed
12 1210 ml per day, 134 ml per feed
13 140 ml per day, 35 ml per feed

Recommended Further Reading

Anaesthesia

Aspinall, V. 2003. *Clinical procedures in veterinary nursing.* Oxford: Butterworth Heinemann.

Hall, L.W. and Clarke, K.W. 1991. *Veterinary anaesthesia.* London: Baillière Tindall.

Lane, D. R. and Cooper, B. 2003. *Veterinary nursing,* 3rd ed. Oxford: Butterworth Heinemann.

Lomas, A., Morgan, A., Allan, L. and Blezard, M. 2004. *How to get through NVQ 3.* Knutsford: PasTest Ltd.

Orpet, H. and Welsh, P. 2002. *Handbook of veterinary nursing.* Oxford: Blackwell Science.

Bandaging

Aspinall, V. 2003. *Clinical procedures in veterinary nursing.* Oxford: Butterworth Heinemann.

Connor, J. and McKerrill, J. 2003. *The Millpledge bandage book.* Retford: Millpledge.

Lane, D. R. and Cooper, B. 2003. *Veterinary nursing,* 3rd ed. Oxford: Butterworth Heinemann.

Orpet, H. and Welsh, P. 2002. *Handbook of veterinary nursing.* Oxford: Blackwell Science.

Fluid Therapy

Aspinall, V. 2003. *Clinical procedures in veterinary nursing.* Oxford: Butterworth Heinemann.

Hotston-Moore, P. 2003. *Fluid therapy for veterinary nurses and technicians.* Amsterdam: Elsevier.

Lane, D. R. and Cooper, B. 2003. *Veterinary nursing,* 3rd ed. Oxford: Butterworth Heinemann.

Orpet, H. and Welsh, P. 2002. *Handbook of veterinary nursing.* Oxford: Blackwell Science.

Laboratory Tests

Aspinall, V. 2003. *Clinical procedures in veterinary nursing.* Oxford: Butterworth Heinemann.

Bush, B. M. 1975. *Veterinary laboratory manual.* Oxford: Heinemann.

Lane, D. R. and Cooper, B. 2003. *Veterinary nursing,* 3rd ed. Oxford: Butterworth Heinemann.

Lomas, A., Morgan, A., Allan, L. and Blezard, M. 2004. *How to get through NVQ 3.* Knutsford: PasTest Ltd.

Orpet, H. and Welsh, P. 2002. *Handbook of veterinary nursing.* Oxford: Blackwell Science.

Medical Nursing

Aspinall, V. 2003. *Clinical procedures in veterinary nursing.* Oxford: Butterworth Heinemann.

Lane, D. R. and Cooper, B. 2003. *Veterinary nursing,* 3rd ed. Oxford: Butterworth Heinemann.

Lomas, A., Morgan, A., Allan, L. and Blezard, M. 2004. *How to get through NVQ 3.* Knutsford: PasTest Ltd.

Orpet, H. and Welsh, P. 2002. *Handbook of veterinary nursing.* Oxford: Blackwell Science.

Radiography

Aspinall, V. 2003. *Clinical procedures in veterinary nursing.* Oxford: Butterworth Heinemann.

Douglas, S.W., Herrtage, M.E. and Williamson, H.D. 1987. *Principles of veterinary radiography*, 4th ed. London: Baillière Tindall.

Easton, S. 2002. *Practical radiography for veterinary nurses.* Oxford: Butterworth Heinemann.

Lane, D. R. and Cooper, B. 2003. *Veterinary nursing*, 3rd ed. Oxford: Butterworth Heinemann.

Lee, R. 1995. *BSAVA manual of small animal diagnostic imaging.* Quedgeley, Gloucestershire: BSAVA.

Lomas, A., Morgan, A., Allan, L. and Blezard, M. 2004. *How to get through NVQ 3.* Knutsford: PasTest Ltd.

Orpet, H. and Welsh, P. 2002. *Handbook of veterinary nursing.* Oxford: Blackwell Science.

Surgical Nursing

Aspinall, V. 2003. *Clinical procedures in veterinary nursing.* Oxford: Butterworth Heinemann.

Atkinson, L.J. and Fortunato, N. 2003. *Operating room technique*, 10th ed. New York: Mosby.

Lane, D. R. and Cooper, B. 2003. *Veterinary nursing*, 3rd ed. Oxford: Butterworth Heinemann.

Orpet, H. and Welsh, P. 2002. *Handbook of veterinary nursing.* Oxford: Blackwell Science.

Useful Addresses

British Small Animal Veterinary Association (BSAVA)
Woodrow House
1 Telford Way
Waterwells Business Park
Quedgeley
Gloucester GL2 4AB
01452 726700

British Veterinary Nursing Association (BVNA)
Suite 11, Shenval House
South Road
Harlow
Essex CM20 2BD
01279 450567

LANTRA
Lantra House
NAC
Kenilworth
Warwickshire CV8 2LG
0845 707 8007
www.lantra.co.uk

Qualifications and Curriculum Authority (QCA)
83 Piccadilly
London W1J 8QA
www.qca.org.uk

Royal College of Veterinary Surgeons (RCVS)
Belgravia House
62–64 Horseferry Road
London SW1P 2AF
0207 222 2001
www.rcvs.org.uk

Scottish Qualification Authority (SQA)
Hanover House
24 Douglas Street
Glasgow G27 N8

Index

A

adhesive bandage, leg 24, 25
Allis tissue forceps 137
ammonium urate crystals 55
anaesthesia 11–17
  quick test (calculations) 17–19
anaesthetic flow rate
  calculation 15–16
  quick test (calculations) 17–19
anatomical directions, for
  radiography 101

B

Babcock's tissue forceps 137
Backhaus towel clip 137
Bain circuit 12, 13
bandaging 21–3
Bard-Parker scalpel handle
  137
basal energy requirement (BER)
  calculations 93–4
  quick test (calculations)
    94–7
BER *see* basal energy requirement
  (BER)
bladder expression 87, 89
blood, packed cell volume (PCV)
  measurement 61–2
blood smear processing 66–8
blood transfusion
  calculations 41–2, 43
  quick test (calculations)
    44–7
bone cutters 138
bone plates 135
bone-holding forceps 138
bowel clamp, Doyen 136
BVA Hip Dysplasia Scheme,
  radiographs for 104–5

C

calcium oxalate dihydrate crystals
  55
carpus, dorsopalmar radiograph
  124–5
caudocranial stifle positioning
  114–15
Certificates in Small Animal
  Veterinary Nursing Theory 3
cervical spine, lateral survey
  radiography 106–7
Cheatle forceps 134, 137
Cheyletiella mite 60
chisel 139
circuit factors 12
circuits, anaesthetic 11–15
closed gloving 131
clothing, protective *see* gloves;
  protective clothing
Co-axial Lack circuit 12
cohesive bandage
  ear 30, 31
  leg 24, 25
compound fracture of the leg,
  bandaging 33–4
conforming bandage
  leg 24, 25
  over immobilising splint 28
  paw 26, 27
contrast, for pneumocystogram
  108
cotton wool, bandaging 24–7
coupage 87, 88
cross-action towel clip 137
crystalloid fluid, requirements
  41–4
crystals, in urine 54–5
Ctenocephalides felis 59
cystine crystals 55

INDEX

D

daily energy requirements,
calculation 77–8
daily fluid requirements,
calculation 41
delivery rate, fluid requirements,
calculation 41
Demodex canis 60
dental explorer 140
dental extraction forceps 140
dental instruments 140
dental probe 140
dental scaler, double-ended 140
diabetes mellitus, management
91–2
dietary requirement, calculation
77–8
dipstick tests, urine 65
disease factor, in daily dietary
requirements 77
dorsal recumbency, in
radiography 104–5
dorsopalmar radiograph, carpus
124–5
dorsoventral thorax positioning
118–19
double-ended dental scaler 140
Doyen bowel clamp 136
draping procedure, sterile trolley
134
dressing scissors 135
drip, intravenous 37–40
drip rate, calculation 41
drug doses
calculations 80–2
quick test (calculations) 83–4
dynamic compression plate 135

E

ear haemorrhage, bandaging 30–1
ectoparasite identification 58–60
effleurage technique 90
endotracheal tubes, in anaesthesia
13, 16–17
examination (day)
arrival for 5–6
examiners 8–9

mitigating circumstances 9
oral questions 7–8
practical tasks 6–7
sections 6–7

F

feeding
basal energy requirements
(BER), calculations 93–4
naso-oesophageal 77–9
Felicola subrostratus 59
Feline Urological Syndrome (FUS)
53
Ferguson angiotribes haemostat
136
Fergusson's bone-holding forceps
138
first aid
compound leg fracture 33–4
immobilising limb splint 28–9
flow rates *see* gas flow rates
fluid therapy 37–44
calculations 41–4
quick test (calculations) 44–7
Foley catheter 85–6
forceps 136, 137
bone-holding 138
dental extraction 140
handling technique 142
forepaw, bandaging post-surgery
26–7
friction massage technique 90

G

gas flow rates, in anaesthesia
15–16, 17–19
Gelpi retractor 138
Gilles needle holder 137
gloves, in the laboratory 53
gloving procedures 131–3
gown donning procedure 129–30
grass-seed, bandaging post-surgical
removal 26–7

H

haematocrit reader 61–2
haemorrhage, ear bandaging 30–1

head bandage   30–1
health and safety   12
  when bandaging   21, 30, 32, 35
  anaesthetic equipment   11–12
  in the laboratory   49
Heath scissors   135
Hip Dysplasia Scheme, radiographs for   104–5
histology sample, packaging   52, 56–7
Hohmann retractor   138
hypostatic pneumonia, prevention   87–8

I
immobilising splint, limb fracture   28–9
instruments, surgical   134–40
  handling   141–2
insulin, use and administration   91–2
intravenous catheters   38
intravenous drip   37–40, 41
intubation   16–17
  equipment   13
Ixodes spp   59

J
Jackson Rees modified Ayres T-piece circuit   12, 14–15
Jacob's chuck   139

K
Kennel Club Hip Dysplasia Scheme, radiographs for   104–5
Kocher and Halstead mosquito   136

L
lab form   57
laboratory techniques   49–52
Lagenbeck retractor   138
Lane forceps   136
Lane tissue forceps   137
lateral lumbar spine   110–11

lateral recumbency positioning
  lateral spine survey   106–7
  lateral tibia radiograph   112–13
  lumbar spine radiograph   110–11
  skull radiograph   120–1
lateral thorax positioning   102–3
leg fracture
  compound, bandaging   33–4
  surgical fixation, bandaging   24–7
Lempert rongeurs   138
limb fracture, immobilising splint   28–9
Linognathus setosus   59
Liston bone-cutters   138
lumbar spine, right lateral survey radiograph   110–11

M
MacPhail's needle holder   137
Magill circuit   12, 14
maintenance requirements, fluid   42–3
Mayo needle holders   136
Mayo scissors   135
medical nursing   73–4
Metzenbaum scissors   135
microscope   50
microscope slides, vernier scales   68–9
microscope use
  ectoparasites   58–60
  urinary sediment   54–5
minute volume, calculation   16
mouth gag, rodent   140

N
naso-oesophageal feeding   77–9
National Vocational Qualification (NVQ)   2–3
needle holders
  Gilles   137
  MacPhail's   137
  Mayo   136

neonates, revival and
    resuscitation 75–6
neuromuscular blocking agents
    16–17
Notoedres cati 60

O
open gloving 132–3
orthopaedic instruments 138–9
orthopaedic screwdriver 139
osteotome 139
Otodectes cynotis 60
owners, communication with
    bandage aftercare 23
    drug dosage 81

P
packed cell volume (PCV),
    measurement 61–2
padding, in ear bandaging 30, 31
Parallel Lack circuit 12, 14
parasites 51
    identification 58–60
paw, bandaging post-surgery
    26–7
PCV *see* packed cell volume (PCV)
periosteal elevator 139
petrissage technique 90
physiotherapy 87–90
plain dressing forceps 136
plantarodorsal radiograph, tarsus
    122–3
plate benders 139
pneumocystogram, right lateral
    108–9
pneumonia (hypostatic),
    prevention 87–8
portfolio completion 2–3
positioning
    for radiography 99
    in physiotherapy 87–8
post-operative bandages
    leg internal fixation 24, 25
    paw grass-seed removal 26,
        27
    support 32
pressure sores, prevention 87, 90

protective clothing
    in the laboratory 49
    in the operating theatre 128,
        129–33

R
radiography 99–101
radius and ulna
    compound fracture, bandaging
        33–4
    fracture 24–7
Rampley's sponge-holding
    forceps 136
rasp 139
refractometer technique, urine
    specific gravity 63–4
retractors 138
revival and resuscitation,
    neonates 75–6
Robert Jones bandage 24–7, 33–4
rodent mouth gag 140
root elevator, dental 140
Royal College of Veterinary
    Surgeons (RCVS) qualifications
        3

S
safety for staff *see* health and safety
sample collection 51
sample packaging 52, 56–7
Sarcoptes scabiei 59
scaler, dental 140
scalpel handle, Bard-Parker 137
scissors 135
    handling technique 141–2
Sherman plate 135
skull, right lateral radiograph
    120–1
specific gravity of urine,
    refractometer technique
        63–4
Spencer Wells forceps 136
spine radiography
    cervical lateral 106–7
    lateral survey 106–7
    lumbar lateral 110–11
splint, limb fracture 28–9

sterile gowning and gloving
    129–33
sterile trolley   134–40
sternal recumbent position   87,
    88
    dorsopalmar carpus   124–5
    plantarodorsal tarsus   122–3
stifle, caudocranial radiograph
    114–15
stirrups, in bandaging   24, 25
struvite crystals   55
subgingival curette   140
surgical instruments   134–40
    handling   141–2
    trolley   134
surgical nursing   127–8
    see also post-operative bandages
suture materials   128, 141

T
T-piece circuit   12, 14–15
tablet bottle and label   81
tarsus, plantarodorsal radiograph
    122–3
theatre nursing   127–8
thoracic bandages   35–6
thoracic radiographs   102–3
    dorsoventral   118–19
    ventrodorsal   116–17
tibia, lateral radiograph   112–13
tidal volume, calculation   16
tissue forceps   137
toe protection
    in leg bandaging   24, 25
    in paw bandaging   26, 27
    with immobilising splint   28
towel clips   137
Travers retractor   138
Treves forceps   136
Trichodectes canis   59

trolley, sterile   134–40
Trombicula autumnalis larva   60
tube feeding   77–9

U
urinary catheterisation   85–6
    for pneumocystogram   108
urine samples
    crystals   51
    processing   63–5
    sediment examination   53–5
    specific gravity   63–4

V
Venables plate   135
ventrodorsal pelvis   105
ventrodorsal thorax   116–17
vernier scales   50, 51
    quick tests (practice)   69–71
    revision notes   68–9
Veterinary Nursing Examination
    5–9
    history of   1–3
veterinary nursing qualifications
    1–3
Vocationally Related Qualifications
    (VRQs)   3
Volkman's scoop   139

W
West retractor   138
whole blood, requirements
    41–4
wound dressing
    leg, post-surgery   24
    paw, post-surgery   26
    under immobilising splint   28

X
X-ray see radiography